The Beginner's Guide to Smoothies

By Kevin J. Finn, Ph.D.

09-May-2020

Eric,

The Threshold Four are bound for great things. This is the start of an adventure. Happy to be working alongside you!

Best,
Kevin

Table of Contents

The Author's Picks 14

Introduction 15

    How to Use This Book 19

Where to Begin? 21

    Essential Kitchen Tools 24

    Optional Kitchen Tools 24

Smoothies, Juices and Whole Fruits and Vegetables 25

    An Easy Formula for Health - Fruits and Vegetables Should Represent Half of Your Diet 26

    What are the Benefits to Juices over Whole Foods? 27

    Smoothies vs Juices-Who Wins? 27

    Fruit Juices and Sugar Level 29

    Which is better - fruit or vegetable juices? 30

    Organic vs. Conventionally Grown 31

    How about Supplements? 37

Antioxidants, Exercise and Sport and Diet 39

    Workout Wonder Juice 40

    Ginger-Pear For the Win 41

Juicer selection 41

What can't be juiced? 46

Order of Operations...48

Juice Fasts 48

Proponents Argue 50

Opponents argue...53

Chemical, Mineral and Nutrient Components-An Introduction......55

Antioxidants..55

Carotenoids...56

Chlorophyll 57

Enzymes 59

Fats and Fatty Acids 59

Fiber 60

Magnesium..61

Polysaccharides 62

Phytonutrients 63

Phytoestrogens 63

Proteins..64

Vitamin C 66

Vitamin K 66

Juicing Ingredients and Description 67

Aloe Vera 67

Apples 67

Avocado 68

Banana 69

Beet 70

Blackberries 71

Blueberries 71

Cantaloupe 72

Cherries 72

Cactus Pear Fruit (Tuna) 73

Coconut 74

Coconut Water 74

Grapes 75

Grapefruit 75

Guava 76

Lemons 76

Limes 77

Lychees 77

Kiwis 78

Mangos 78

Oranges..78

Passion Fruit 79

Papayas..80

Pears..80

Persimmons...81

Pineapple...81

Pomegranate 82

Starfruit...83

Strawberries 83

Raspberries..84

Watermelon...84

Vegetables 84

Cactus (Nopales) 84

Carrots 85

Celery 85

Cucumber..86

Dandelion Greens..86

Fennel...87

Kale 88

Peppers (Bell, Chili) 88

Radishes..89

Spinach 90

Sweet Potato...91

Tofu (Soy) 91

Tomato..92

Wheatgrass..92

Herbs, Spices & Roots...93

Basil...93

Cayenne Pepper 94

Cilantro...94

Cinnamon...95

Garlic...95

Ginger 96

Turmeric 97

Green Smoothies 98

What Makes a Green Smoothie? 99

The pH Effect 101

Lemon and Water 102

Original Green Smoothie 103

Cactus Smoothie 104

Cleveland Clinic Green Grape Smoothie Recipe 105

Luminous Skin Smoothie 106

Banana Blueberry 106

Creamy Green Banana Smoothie 107

Beet Green Smoothie 107

Guava Green 108

Green Pear Smoothie 108

Melon Kale 109

Coconut Clementine Green Smoothie 109

Dandelion Green Smoothie 110

Kiwi Melon Green Smoothie 110

Shauna's Carrot Cake Smoothie 111

Fruit Smoothies 112

Mango Berry 112

Watermelon Cooler 113

Blue Melon 114

Super Berry 114

Orange-Cantaloupe...........115

Mango-Coconut...........115

Peach Berry 116

Beet & Berry 116

Mango Papaya Morning Start 117

Pineapple-Kiwi-Coconut...........117

Berry Coconut Water Smoothie...........118

Pomegranate Mango...........118

Jam Master Juice (aka Joseph Persimmons)...........119

Passion Fruit Watermelon...........120

Guava Fruit 121

Guava Mango 121

Mango Beet 122

Lychee-Pineapple Cooler 122

Berry Fiber...........123

Mango Plum...........123

Cactus Pear Strawberry Cooler 124

Blueberry-Pear Smoothie 124

Clementine-Strawberry 125

Tropical Beet 125

Guava Strawberry Green Tea 126

Banana Strawberry Kiwi 126

Mango Banana Kiwi....................127

Fall Strawberry Persimmon 127

Aloevita Tropical Smoothie 128

Fall Strawberry Persimmon Smoothie....................129

Fresh Juices....................129

Cilantro-Celery-Ginger....................129

Orange-Pineapple-Celery-Carrot....................130

Orange Dreamsicle....................130

Beet-Carrot-Pineapple 131

Mango Coconut Pineapple....................132

Pomegranate-Lime....................132

Vitamin C Supercharge 133

Cucumber-Apple....................133

Pomegranate Kiwi..134

Beet Carrot Apple..134

Persimmon-Kiwi-Apple 134

Purple Viking...135

Orange Sunrise 135

Peach Orange Delight..136

Apple Berry Lemonade 137

The Eye Doctor 137

Beet Carrot Apple Celery 138

Starfruit Sorpresa 138

Cactus Pear Cooler...139

Cactus Kiwi Orange 139

Cactus Sunrise 140

Grapefruit Nectarine..141

Pomegranate Grape Juice 141

Grape Strawberry Juice 141

Beet-Grapefruit-Orange..142

Sweet Beet 142

Clementine-Apple...142

Beet Mixture...143

Spicy Hot V10 Vegetable Juice 144

Captain Chlorophyll 145

Tart Berry Currant..146

Top Tummy 146

Wheatgrass-Mango-Cactus Pear 147

Green Liver Tonic...147

Morning Green Energy...148

Simple Cherry Juice 148

Total Health Cleanser 148

Detoxifying Radish Blend 149

Vegetable Cleanser...150

Green Orange Fennel Juice 150

Spicy Fennel Beet 150

Pineapple Carrot Super Root....................................151

Super Beet Cleanser 151

Fennel-Beet...152

Cucumber Lemon Cooler...152

Cucumber Beet 153

Orange Vegetable Juice 153

Pineapple Cucumber-Guava 153

Beet Grapefruit 154

Sweet Orange Sunrise..154

Fennel Radish Cleanser 154

Heart Healer..155

Inflammation Fighter...156

Purple Inflammation Fighter 156

Salsa in a Glass...157

Mexican Gazpacho 157

Cucumber, Carrot and Beet 158

Garden Variety[66]...158

Cold Combat...158

Island Punch 159

Super Green Zinger..159

Natural Baby Foods 160

Purees...161

Apricots 161

Juices 161

    Carrot Juice...161

    Apple Juice 162

Smoothies 162

    Apple Cinnamon 163

    Orange Basil 163

    Cherry Berry 163

    Banana Smoothie 164

    Mango Lassi Smoothie...164

    Strawberry Smoothie 164

    Banana-Berry Treat 164

  About the Author 165

References 166

The Author's Picks

This is likely the first section you're reading, but it is the last that I've written. If you are a person of action like myself, you may want to charge into the kitchen and get started on your new endeavor right away. So here is what I offer. If you read **nothing** other than these first two pages, I want to make the price of this book worth it to you. I sincerely hope you take the time to read about the healthy fruits and vegetables, a bit of biochemistry and tricks and tips for best juicing and smoothie preparation. But if nothing else, I want you to take away my top 10 juices and smoothies. I hope you enjoy and share!

Table 1: Kevin's Top Ten Juices and Smoothies

Top Smoothies	Top Juices
Original Green Smoothie 1 cup orange juice ½ cup pineapple 1 cup spinach 1 kale leaf 1 green apple 1 stalk celery 3 slices ginger	**Orange Dreamsicle** 1 green apple 1 stalk celery 1 orange, peeled 1 pear 1 sweet potato ½ tsp fresh ginger
Blue Melon 2 cups watermelon 1 cup blueberries ½ cup crushed ice	**Cucumber, Carrot and Beet** 3 carrots ½ cucumber ½ beet with greens

Banana Strawberry Kiwi	Beet Carrot Apple
8 oz orange juice	3 oz beet juice
½ banana	3 oz carrot juice
2 kiwis	3 oz apple juice
3 oz strawberries	1 tsp shaved ginger
½ cup ice	
Aloevita Tropical Smoothie	**Cold Combat**
8 oz frozen pineapple chunks	1 white grapefruit
1 large ripe mango, peeled and deseeded	1 cup pineapple
	2 Bartlett pears
1 cup of fresh Thai coconut water	1 tsp ginger, grated.
2 oz fresh Thai coconut flesh	
½ cup aloe vera pulp	
Blueberry-Pear Smoothie	**Heart Healer**
½ cup chilled water	1 cucumber
8 oz blueberries	1 pear
3 oz pineapple (or more for sweeter taste)	Handful of mint leaves
	1 fennel bulb and stalks
1 oz spinach	1 celery stalk
1 pear	Makes 12 oz
3 oz plain yogurt	
½ cup crushed ice	

Introduction

Never in history have we been so busy, stretched so thinly and have so many demands placed on our time. As work-life equilibrium tips out of balance, diet is one of the first casualties-too often with devastating results.

Every five years, the United States Dietary Guidelines Advisory Committee (DGAC), a joint scientific committee composed of the U.S. Department of Agriculture and the Department of Health and Human Services issues a scientific report to help Americans make informed choices about diet and health. The 2015 draft Scientific Report from this advisory board concluded that approximately 117 million American adults have "one or more preventable, chronic diseases that are related to poor quality dietary patterns and physical inactivity, including cardiovascular disease, hypertension, type 2 diabetes and diet related cancers".[1] As the study goes on to report, dietary problems are associated with an American diet low in vegetables, fruit and whole grain while high in saturated fats, sugars and calories. Vitamin C, iron, vitamin A and calcium were underrepresented in the typical American diet.

An impressive body of work provides evidentiary connection between our diets and our physical and mental health. Documentaries such as "Forks over Knives" based on seminal the China Study by Dr. T. Colin Campbell and clinical evidence from cardiologist Dr. Caldwell Essylsten, Jr. have done well to raise the visibility of these relationships and impress on us the benefits of adopting a whole foods plant-based diet. The realization that our diets are inextricably linked to our well-being is no longer in question. The human body evolved to its present state in balance with nature when meat was scarce, vegetables were not frozen, salt was difficult to obtain, and the day-to-day rigor of life kept our bodies far more active state. In comparison to our ancestors, we consume too many calories, a large portion of which are sugars or fats and far too few vegetables and fruits.

Joe Cross, author of *The Reboot with Joe Juice Diet*, explains the distinction between macronutrients and micronutrients and the importance of consuming the correct balance of the two for good overall health. Macronutrients include proteins, carbohydrates and fats, which are readily obtained from daily products, meats and processed foods. The typical Western diet tends to be heavy on macronutrient intake. Micronutrients, however, are the essential phyto (plant) nutrients, vitamins, enzymes and minerals which are so critical to warding off disease and maintaining the body's optimal performance. The Harvard Health Publishing[2] group emphasizes the importance of micronutrients in maintenance of brain, skin, nerve, blood circulation. There are nearly 30 vitamins and minerals which are "essential", meaning that the body cannot itself manufacture these and that they must be sourced from the foods we eat. There is certainly a link between disease prevention, micronutrient consumption and the immune system. Immune boosting micronutrients include vitamin B_6, vitamin C, vitamin E, magnesium and zinc are best obtained from a well-rounded diet including many fruits and vegetables.

Now that we understand the importance of a well-balanced diet, how do we address this in practice. Life's inertia makes it difficult to break with poor eating habits, establish new routines and regain control over our health. People need to understand choices and be offered an alternative. Moreover, the alternative must be enjoyable, relatively easy and one which enjoys measurable benefits. Like all new habits, the shift to adopting a healthy habit must be manageable and gradual. I believe the recipes contained in this book offer exactly that- a quick start, low barrier entry into a new and healthful diet.

I was intrigued to learn that, when an acquaintance suffered a heart attack in 2012, upon recovery the doctor prescribed a plant-based diet, including a green smoothie breakfast each morning. As it is with automobiles, homes, gadgets and most things in life, it is far easiest to maintain than to repair or replace. And with this philosophy in mind, I aimed to maintain my health with a daily routine of a green smoothie breakfast.

The green smoothie I was introduced to was one of endless varieties which are enjoyed by many as a tool to lower cholesterol, lose weight, maintain good heart health and reverse the health problems. When my father was diagnosed with cancer in 2014, we looked to nutrition and dietary methods to supplement the chemotherapeutic and radiation treatment he received. Incidentally, I found a very similar "green smoothie" offered in the Cleveland Clinic's Cancer health publication. Through this research, I learned that many cancer survivors have attributed their success, at least in part, to dietary changes in combination with traditional cancer treatments. For many, the nutritional changes embraced in the course of treatment were adopted as part of a new healthy lifestyle. These changes were transformational for many so much so, that several survivors credit their cancer with spurring on overdue shifts in lifestyle.

Fresh juices invigorate, energize, cleanse and maintain. The variety of brews, through various combinations of ingredients, is endless and the benefits span a similar spectrum. We have found juicing to be an adventure. Each market, each season provides a new collection of ingredients. We are constantly challenged to expand our repertoire, incorporating new fruits, herbs, vegetables and spices to provide both healthful and appetizing concoctions.

How to Use This Book

This book is for everyone who wants to experience the transformation that fresh, homemade and preservative free juices can provide. As a juicing enthusiast, I have read several books on juicing and follow many great online blogs for sharing recipes and recounting stories of personal transformation. One humorous blogger admitted he often wandered around the market, wondering, "Can I juice that?" With a few notable exceptions, the answer is usually, "Yes!". This became the working title of my juicing blog http://canijuiceit.wordpress.com, which served as the foundation for the present work.

Where to begin? I understand that selection of fruits and choosing combinations to blend may be a bit daunting in the beginning. Not to worry. This edition includes an introduction to the most common fruits, vegetables and herbs for use in fresh juices. I intentionally placed the alphabetized listing of fruits, vegetables and components at the beginning to familiarize the reader with the "characters" in the book and their role in keeping us healthy.

The *Quick Tips* sections provide practical suggestions from storage recommendations to extend the lifetime of your ingredients to instructions on purchase and preparation of juicing ingredients. For those thirsting to know more about the principal chemical constituents of the ingredients and some of their putative mechanisms of action, a reference table is provided in Appendix 1.

It is also recognized that most juices for **children** found in the grocery store contain mostly processed juices and contain large amounts of sugar. A key initiative is to help teach children the benefits of eating fruits and vegetables while appealing to their tastes. Many of these recipes are kid-friendly, having been rigorously tested in our own laboratory (my sister's and brother-in-law's kitchen) with real kids. I welcome your feedback as these experiments are conducted in your own home.

Finally, as an extension to the section on children's smoothies and juices, I offer a section on the preparation of baby foods in combination with the juicer. We believe that the satisfaction of preparing your child's first foods from natural ingredients in your own kitchen will be unmatched. Not only can you prepare the foods in combinations and quantities serving your child's tastes and needs, these foods contain no preservatives and provide a full spectrum of healthful variety. The flexibility and speed of preparation will save you time and money.

Though all the juices and smoothies contain a potent mixture of vitamins, minerals, antioxidants and cancer-fighting power, those seeking a certain benefit (weight loss, energy, etc.) will find the classification useful. The benefits of certain chilies are also identified and explained. Those recipes having a spicy chili component are denoted with the symbol .

Through practice, I have generated a menu of healthy smoothie options employing both a simple blender and a masticating juicer. Recipes for both methods are offered befitting your schedule and taste. Use what is fresh and offered at your grocer or farmer's market according to season in your area. Feel free to make substitutions, create your own favorites and let your taste (and your families) be the guide.

Where to Begin?

"Think big, start small, act now" - Barnabas Suebu, governor of the Indonesian province of Papua

Paradigm shifts in lifestyle and health will inevitably start small. Charles Duhigg's best-selling book, "The Power of Habit" impresses on us how central habit is to evoking change in behavior, irrespective of the behavior we wish to change. Mr. Duhigg speaks of "transformational habits"; small, perhaps seemingly inconsequential changes in our actions which tend toward a domino effect in behavioral patterns. Adopting juices and smoothies into my diet has become such a transformational habit. Fresh juices and smoothies invigorate me, which gives me energy to exercise. The exercise lowers my stress level and, in turn, provides me focus and energy to accomplish my goals for the day, which, in turn, gives me a sense of well-being. The exercise has the added benefit of allowing me to sleep better so that I am well-rested and can begin the next day feeling fresh and recharged. Additionally, being intentional about what you put into your morning smoothie will tend to create an enhanced awareness about your diet, in general. Such is the power of a transformational habit. Here are a few ways to begin to get engaged in this new habit:

1) Find a smoothie shop to sample flavors and allow your body to get accustomed. Many high-end grocery stores are popping up which offer in-store smoothies or fresh juices.

2) If you are hesitant to make the investment in a juicer, begin by introducing some blended smoothies into your diet. Begin with a simple green smoothie and try to have this every day for a week, or better still, for 30 days.

3) Look up a recipe or two before going to the grocery store. Having everything you need makes it more likely to make your juice or smoothie.

4) Seek out a new grocery store or farmer's market. See what's in season and fresh. If you have the opportunity, an Asian or Latin American market promises adventure and will allow you access to coconuts, aloe, mangos, guava, lychees, cactus and many other fruits and vegetables to spice up your smoothies.

5) Establish a dedicated space for your juicer or blender in your kitchen. Easy access to your essential tools will lower the resistance to getting in a routine.

6) Plenty of great resources are available for recipes, tips and advice. Take advantage of the popularity of the juicer's blogs on the internet. Additionally, many great references are provided in the Reference section.

The recipes collected in this book are far more than you'll need to settle into a routine of healthy juicing and smoothie intake. If you find 10 smoothie and juice recipes you enjoy, you'll be well on your journey to a healthier lifestyle. This keeps the shopping list simpler and will make for easier daily routine. In less time that it takes to make a hot breakfast, you could be enjoying a healthy smoothie to carry you through a busy morning.

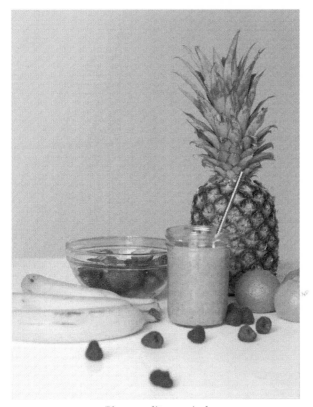

Photo credit: rawpixel

Essential Kitchen Tools

I've found the following to be indispensable tools for preparing juices and smoothies:

Blender

Juicer

Sharp knives

Vegetable peeler/scrubber

Easy to wash, non-staining cutting boards

Selection of measuring cups

Selection of measuring spoons

Rasp or Zester (for grating ginger and cinnamon)

Orange/lime squeezer

Strainer for washing berries

Optional Kitchen Tools

The following are optional, but helpful additions to your arsenal depending on your needs for storage:

- *Vacuum storage containers for juice (such as Vacucraft®)*

- *Sealable freezer bags or containers*

- *Squeasy Snacker® reusable silicone pouch for storage and dispensing children's juices and smoothies*

- *Kitchen scale*

Smoothies, Juices and Whole Fruits and Vegetables

In natural foods, Nature has provided the perfect balance of energy, protective enzymes, immune-boosters and protein building blocks. What is the origin of these components? How do they interact? Scientists and nutritionists have dedicated years of research and millions of dollars to the quest for dissecting our foods into chemical constituents to understand their makeup and potential for healthful benefit. Unfortunately, our scientific efforts have perhaps done more to confound the issue and thereby confuse the public. It is with little wonder that people, frustrated with receiving conflicting information, throw up their hands and resolve to eat simply what they enjoy. What is the source of this conflict and why can't scientists agree on the scientific data? The key difficulty associated with these well-intentioned scientific endeavors lies in decoupling the synergistic properties of the chemical components working in cooperation in whole foods. The 2010 DGAC report noted "that it is often not possible to separate the effects of individual nutrients and foods, and that the totality of diet—the combinations and quantities in which foods and nutrients are consumed—may have synergistic and cumulative effects on health and disease."

An Easy Formula for Health - Fruits and Vegetables Should Represent Half of Your Diet

According to the United States Department of Agriculture (USDA)[3] we should be consuming about 5-9 servings of a variety of fruits and vegetables per day. Very simply, about *half* of the foods you eat should be plants-and this is a conservative estimate. The USDA's "choose my plate" initiative[4] offers practical guidance for maintaining a healthy diet. The colorful logo (**Figure 1**) provides an easy visual directive for the relative amount of fruits and vegetables to be consumed.

Figure 1: The USDA's ChooseMyPlate.gov Logo

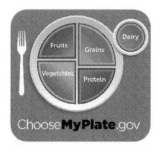

Many experts advocate a diet based completely on plants and there is a growing mountain of data of supporting the associated benefits. The USDA, in its 2010 Report of the Dietary Guidelines Committee,[5] recommends to "shift food intake patterns to a **more plant-based diet that emphasizes vegetables**, cooked dry beans and peas, **fruits**, whole grains, nuts, and seeds." (emphasis mine).

What are the Benefits to Juices over Whole Foods?

One of the most commonly asked questions is: "Why juice foods when they can simply be eaten?" The first reason is that the amount of fruits and vegetables per unit volume for smoothies and juices is appreciably higher. This translates into a higher nutritional content per glass. It would practically take all day to eat the amount of produce in a single 8 oz serving of juice. In other words, smoothies and juices pack a bigger punch per glass and allow one to "eat" the rainbow of fruits and vegetables without having to spend the time and energy eating the individual whole foods. Secondly, when mixed in the right proportions, the individual components complement one another to provide an excellent balance of taste, not to mention its nutritional benefit. Of course, whole foods should always remain the principal part of the diet, but a juice or smoothie can provide a bit of supplemental nutrition or serve as a healthy snack or meal replacement. Lastly, juicing allows us to combine those fruits, vegetables and roots into our diet which have been used in traditional medicine for years without having to eat them raw or cook them (fennel and ginger come to mind). Some of these foods would simply be too difficult or powerful to eat as whole foods and cooking can destroy some powerful enzymes and, in some cases, erode the nutritional benefit.

Smoothies vs Juices-Who Wins?

Smoothies offer an advantage over juices in that they can be simply made in a blender or mixed with ice for a refreshing treat. Depending on your equipment, blending usually requires less effort in preparation and clean-up relative to a juicing machine. Smoothies are the original healthy "fast food". Finally, the added fiber contained in the smoothie relative to a juiced product is more filling and the fiber slows the release of sugars into the blood stream. I prefer smoothies in the morning, often substituting fresh juices for store-bought juices. By having smoothie each morning, I am encouraged to have not only breakfast, but a healthy one, at that. The action of blending a smoothie serves to tear down the fibrous material in the fruit, allowing it to be more easily processed by the body. This is one of the reasons it is easier to eat a smoothie containing a variety of fruits or vegetables rather than the same amount of whole foods (**Figure 2**). A juicer, however, separates the bulk of the fiber from the juice and liquid. The nutrients are more easily absorbed into the system when they are concentrated in the juices and separated from the fiber.

Figure 2-Fiber Spectrum

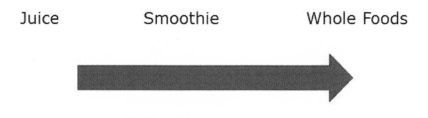

But wait-isn't fiber the good stuff? Fiber *is* good, and juices provide a high content of soluble fiber, the type associated with lowering cholesterol and stabilizing blood sugar levels. For those of us who have sensitive digestive systems, it may be easier to drink juices to avoid taxing the system in processing a large amount of insoluble fiber. The juicer is designed to crush the fruit or vegetable and press out all the liquid containing valuable nutrients and minerals.

The juicer concentrates these nutrients for rapid adsorption into the body. Note that this phenomenon also leads to rapid adsorption of the food sugars and may be associated with an energy "spike". Blending fresh juices into a smoothie will slow the absorption and provide a more even uptake of the fruit sugars.

Fruit Juices and Sugar Level

Recently I read about a diet based on elimination of fruits. The reasoning goes that fruits are simply composed mainly of sugar and water. Before we throw the baby out with the bathwater, let us remember that in addition to water and sugar, fruits are brimming with vital micronutrients, antioxidants and minerals. The synergy of the antioxidants and nutrients is not to be underestimated. It is true that many fruit juices contain natural sugars, which raise blood sugar levels and can result in weight gain if drunk in excess. It is also recognized that modern fruit growers can produce fruits which are far higher in natural sugar than the wild varieties through hybridization[17]. An excessive amount of sugar may disrupt the levels of hormones regulating blood sugar, such as insulin and glucagon. A blood sugar spike can be countered by diluting natural juices with equal parts water to cut the sweetness. Vegetable juices, in general, contain much less sugar and are more suited to a weight loss juice regime.

Jaclyn London, M.S., R.D., a senior dietician at Mount Sinai Hospital in New York City recently shed some light on the topic of juicing and weight gain in the April 24th, 2014 Women's Health magazine. She says that there is a risk of weight gain through juicing if the macronutrients like fats and proteins are missing from the juice. Juices containing the sugars, but without the fiber and protein, can leave us feeling hungry. If we satisfy this hunger with high calorie meals, then weight gain can result. A morning green smoothie should contain around 5 g of fiber, 6 g protein and fall in the range of 200-300 calories to fill you up. I find that adding oatmeal, chia seeds or a little protein powder can help balance the green smoothie. The addition of avocado or yogurt or even tofu slices does the trick for others. Ms. London recommends a lighter, 100 calories or less green smoothie for an on-the-go snack.

Additionally, the fiber can offset some of the blood sugar spike associated with carbohydrate-rich juices. Those combating cancer should be particularly conscious of their sugar intake, as sugars may compromise the natural immune system and provide a food source for rapidly dividing cancer cells. (Refer to Green Smoothies Section).

Which is better - fruit or vegetable juices?

While fruit juices offer provide a natural and great-tasting entry into the juicing arena, they should be properly balanced with green vegetable juices. Diabetics and those keenly monitoring glucose levels should be aware of the relatively high sugar content of not only fruit juices, but also carbohydrate-rich vegetables such as beets and carrots. I tend to supplement vegetable juices with healthy sources of protein and fats when used as a meal replacement. The Green Smoothie section provides such recipes including avocados, tofu or chia seeds as supplement.

In short, incorporate both fruit and vegetable juices into your diet to reap the maximum benefit. The ingredients section highlights an impressive range of benefits, many of which seem to be shared by both fruits and vegetables. For example, both fennel and papaya are excellent ingredients to support good digestive health, while cucumbers and kale are associated with maintenance of good bone and skin health. Rotation of both fruits and vegetables into your diet would seem the best method for avoiding too much of any one thing while enjoying the maximum nutritional benefit.

Monica Reinagel, MS, LD/N, CNS is a board-certified, licensed nutritionist and professionally trained chef offers these well-advised tips for juicing. In her "Nutrition Diva" blog[6], Ms. Reinagel responds to a reader's query about whether drinking 4-5 16 oz serving of fresh fruit/vegetable juice mixtures each day was healthy with respect to intake of sugar and antioxidants. Juicing fruits such as oranges, mango or high-carbohydrate vegetables such as carrots and beets every few hours can result in periodic spikes in blood sugar. She goes on to point out the juices are not complete meals in that they lack essential fatty acids, are low in protein and fiber. In summary, Ms. Reinagel suggests that juices be consumed in moderation in conjunction with other foods for a more balanced diet. Combining juice with a high energy workout routine will help to counter the sugar spike. Finally, she suggests making "whole juice", (i.e. smoothie), which retains the fiber. Note that the Green Smoothie Section contains several recipes which retain not only fiber but offer supplemental ingredients to increase the essential fatty acid and protein content.

Organic vs. Conventionally Grown

Nearly every grocery store has a section devoted to organic produce and organic only stores are on the rise. The supply follows demand as consumers are now more aware than ever about what chemicals they may be unknowingly ingesting. But what is "organic agriculture" and how does it differ from traditional methods of farming? The USDA defines organic agriculture as producing "products that preserve the environment and avoid most synthetic materials, such as pesticides and antibiotics." The USDA put forth standards, which have been promulgated into law by US Congress via the Organic Foods Production Act, delineating methods for farming practices governing soil and water quality, pest control, and materials which may be used. All farms selling products under the "certified organic" rubric must undergo certification, entailing inspection and submission of a plan (a comprehensive control strategy) to an authorized accreditation body on a yearly basis. The certification entails rigorous inspection of farms, the processing facilities and maintenance of detailed documented records of soil and water pesticide testing which is evaluated against Regulatory standards. This extra effort seems to pay off in over $35 billion of growing revenue for certified organic products. But, we consumers are demanding to know whether the benefits gleaned from organic produce justify its substantially higher cost? Importantly, what are the downsides of choosing conventional produce and products, which may be found for half the price of their organic counterparts?

The debate centers on the relative level of two key parameters: nutrient content and relative level of residual pesticides. The aim of science is to substantiate a measurable and statistically significant difference between tested groups. Among the most cited (and

©2018 Kevin Finn

contended) publications on the topic is a comprehensive meta-analysis undertaken in 2012 by Stanford researchers Dena Bravata, M.D. and Crystal Smith-Spangler, M. D[7]. These researchers combed through thousands of papers to whittle down the analysis to 17 published clinical trials and 223 further studies associated with comparing relative content of nutrients or toxins, such as pesticide, fungal or bacterial contaminants in dairy, meat, fruits, vegetables, grains, poultry and eggs. No longitudinal human studies were included in the analysis; the longest trial involving humans was only up to two days. The summary concluded that little significant differences were found in the comparison of nutrients found in traditional and organic products. Case closed, then? Maybe not. First, it is important to understand that, drawing conclusions from analysis of more than 230 studies is a tricky business. And, in the case of fruits and vegetables, nutritional content is also impacted by the freshness of the products.

Other more focused studies paint different picture. A recent study has demonstrated in a group of 40 California children that urine samples[8] collected during consumption periods of organic foods show significantly lower differences in pesticide and related compounds associated with consumption of organic foods. It should be noted, however, that in some cases levels of pesticides were indistinguishable between the two groups. Another confounding factor is that pesticides are used around the home, so that we are generally exposed to some basal level of background pesticide apart from the foods we ingest. It is clear, however, that pesticide exposure should be minimized as many pesticides are demonstrated to be carcinogenic.

In her book, The Juice Lady's Remedies for Stress and Adrenal Failure, "Juice Lady" Cherie Calbom cites a 2007 study which focuses on comparison of flavonoid (an antioxidant) in organic and non-organic tomatoes over a ten-year horizon. The study concluded that the flavonoid content is approximately doubled in the organic group. Flavonoids have been linked to cholesterol regulation and overall cardiovascular protection.

Other studies, such as a Johns Hopkins Ph.D. dissertation, have found that if you are able, shop at farmer's markets for the freshest produce, whether conventional or organic. Again, Cherie Calbom lends sage advice in encouraging shoppers to purchase from local farmers markets. Many of the local farmers cannot claim organic if they haven't registered as such but may be adhering to traditional farming techniques and steer clear of pesticides and chemical fertilizers as part of their standard practice.

"Food miles" is recently introduced term describing the distance food travels from its cultivation to our plates and some argue that the "where" food is grown is more important than "how". Intuitively, we can imagine that food traveling over a longer distance has more opportunity to collect carbon emissions. Additionally, purchase of locally grown produce, as from a farmer's market, affords one the opportunity to speak directly with the grower about the methods used.

The nutritional question of the product aside, organic farming raises the bar for responsible use of land and may prevent undue environmental damage through release of pesticides. The researchers reported that the level of pesticides in conventional foods tipped higher by about 30%, but the maximum threshold was not reached in either group. Again, variance across many study groups is expected, but, in general less pesticides in our foods is good. The notion that organic farming practices are healthier for the farm workers and the environment leaves little doubt. In this respect, it may be a clearer choice for some.

Each year, the Environmental Working Group sifts through over USDA data on pesticide testing of thousands of samples of produce and distills the data set down to a ranking of the pesticide levels of the 48 most commonly consumed fruits and vegetables. From this data set two groups emerge: a "Clean 15[9]", a collection having the lowest amount of pesticide residue and a "dirty dozen", whose members have demonstrated the highest level of pesticide contaminants. The clean 15 for 2018 are report in **Table 2**.

Table 2: The Clean 15 of 2018 as reported by the Environmental Working Group

- Avocado
- Pineapple
- Kiwi
- Papaya
- Mango
- Honeydew Melon
- Cauliflower
- Sweet corn
- Cabbage
- Onions
- Cantaloupe
- Asparagus
- Eggplant
- Cauliflower
- Sweet peas (frozen)

At the opposite end of the spectrum lie the so-called "dirty dozen"[10], the 12 produce members having, as of the 2018 report, the highest level of pesticides as reported by the Environmental Working Group. To give a sense of the span of the study, in 2013, the USDA noted 165 different types of pesticides in a sample of thousands of fruits and vegetables tested. In addition to the 12 dirty dozen shown in **Table 3**, the EWG has recently added a "plus" group comprising produce having highly toxic pesticides, but otherwise do not adhere to the traditional criteria normally characterized by the dirty dozen. The 2018 report assigns hot (chili) peppers to the plus category for their harboring an insecticide found to be highly toxic to the nervous system. Above all, chili peppers should be replaced by organically grown analogues.

Table 3: The Environmental Working Group's 2018 Shopper's Guide to Pesticides in Produce™

• Strawberries	• Grapes	• Tomatoes
• Spinach	• Peaches	• Celery
• Nectarines	• Cherries	• Sweet Bell Peppers
• Apples	• Pears	
		• Potatoes

The group has proposed that consumers who switch to purchasing organic for the dirty dozen may reduce risk of pesticide exposure by over 80% a factor well worthy of note. For us shoppers on a budget, this relatively simple substitution can ensure that we make the most impactful choice where pesticide contamination is concerned.

How about Supplements?

The prevalence of supplements in the US market has virtually exploded since the 1994 Dietary Supplement Health and Education Act, a repositioning which effectively downgraded dietary supplements from the more highly regulated food status to their non-food supplement characterization.

In this same year, the New England Journal of Medicine[11] published findings from a joint study from the National Institutes of Health and Wellness in Finland and the National Cancer Institute involving over 29,000 male smokers from Finland who were prescribed α-tocopherol (vitamin E) or B-carotene supplements or placebo for 5-8 years until close of the study.

Surprisingly, the population of those given the supplement was found a higher incidence of cancer among the participants taking B-carotene supplements. The study highlights an important-though not unique-example of the difficulty in establishing evidence that the effects of a supplement are independent from other factors, such as trace minerals, antioxidants or other yet to be identified entities in the natural source. How is it that an antioxidant and compound in carrots, thought to impart cancer protection, could exert a negative effect? One can imagine the challenge associated with separating the behavior of a compound in combination with hundreds of other compounds and minerals in its natural source with that taken as a supplement. The effects are likely to be different and it is a formidable task to determine the origin of the difference draw conclusions. Certain supplements are clearly beneficial, such as folic acid for pregnant mothers and vitamin D for populations receiving little natural sunlight in the winter season. The medical community itself, seems somewhat divided on the utility of supplements. It is generally understood that the nutrients are best obtained in their natural form through consumption of foods. The benefits associated with the fruits, vegetables and herbs outlined in this book are based on the synergistic effects of using the whole food. The inability to provide direct evidence of certain chemicals operating in isolation does not mean that we do not reap their benefits in whole foods and juices. I am not suggesting that we do away with supplements; my doctor prescribes me vitamin D supplements to maintain good health over the long Chicago winter. I am merely making the point that, when possible, it is best to derive nutrients from their natural sources.

Antioxidants, Exercise and Sport and Diet

Aerobic exercise, better known as "cardio" in recent years offers tremendous benefit for overall physical as well as emotional well-being. How do you know you are getting a good cardio workout? Your heart is beating quickly, and you are perspiring. Your breathing accelerates, allowing your strained lungs to take in extra oxygen and relay O_2 to your tightened muscles. If you can sustain this for more than a few minutes, you are engaging in an aerobic exercise. The wonder of it is that your heart, lungs and muscles adapt to the stain and will ultimately become stronger for it. It is well-known that the oxidative processes associated with exercise produce free radicals (reactive oxygen species), and the widely-held view was that antioxidants were needed post-training to repair damage sustained by the reactive oxidative species. Very often, supplements of antioxidants vitamin C and vitamin E were given to athletes with the intent to scavenge damaging oxygen species with the aid of antioxidants. However, recent scientific studies[12] have demonstrated that no statistical link exists between antioxidant supplementation and reduced recovery time, reduced soreness and increased muscle mass. In short, it is not necessary (and in some cases, counterproductive) to ingest antioxidant supplements post-workout. Instead, Dr. Scott Powers at the University of Florida recommends a well-balanced diet with fruits and vegetables. Juices can play an important role as part of this well-balanced diet and support the processes at work in the athlete. Muscle building, blood circulation, fat breakdown and glucose conversion are all central to support a good cardio workout.

Protein building is essential for healthy response to exercise; a green smoothie or juice can provide a good source of natural protein and the leafy greens in the smoothie or juice contain high amounts of magnesium, which is critical for the body's ability to synthesize proteins and prevent excess fat storage. Carrot juice, which is high in beta carotene, is also known to support oxygenation of the blood, brain and body tissues. Sixteen oz of fresh carrot juice supplies as much protein as a piece of tofu or chicken wing.[13] Finally, the trace mineral chromium is known to increase uptake of glucose, which in turn facilitate blood circulation and is central in building muscle, burning fat and converting energy. Beets are an excellent source of glucose and magnesium. Ginger is known to have anti-inflammatory benefits and can aid in muscle soreness.

Workout Wonder Juice

1 red beet, peeled

4-5 kale leaves or -1/2 cup spinach

1 green apple

6 carrots, peeled

1 in fresh ginger, peeled

2 stalks celery

Introduce each ingredient into the juicer in the order given. Add 2-3 ice cubes

Ginger-Pear For the Win

Recently, Prevention magazine devoted a section to post-workout smoothies, with an emphasis on protein, fiber, antioxidants[14]. The author cited gingerols, a group of compounds derived from fresh ginger, as "potent anti-inflammatories that speed recovery time." Skip the creatine and muscle milk; here is a green smoothie variant offered as a post-workout drink.

½ cup vanilla Greek yogurt

1 ripe pear, cored and cut into large chunks

1 c pear juice or coconut water

½-inch chunk of fresh ginger root or ⅛ tsp dried ground ginger

2 cups baby spinach leaves

1 Tbsp ground flaxseed

½ cup ice cubes

Juicer selection

As any shopper is bound to notice, there is a wide range of prices, sizes and functions associated with juicers on the market. Luckily, several great resources are published. The professionals at Reviews.com have assembled a comprehensive and unbiased review of some of the key characteristics and considerations for juicers, having probed the spectrum from ergonomics to juice output. Here is a direct link to their review: **https://www.reviews.com/juicer/**.

The following section provides my brief overview of the elements one should consider in selecting a juicer. Among the first considerations should be the type of material to be processed. Many juicers are better suited to a specific task and no one single type is capable of processing everything with the same efficiency. For example, certain juicers are more adept at harvesting juices from fruits and vegetables rather than extracting juices from leafy greens. The balance of speed and extraction of nutritional content must also be considered. Juicers operating at high revolutions per minute (rpm) will impart higher friction and attendant heat, and thereby lower the nutrient value of the resulting juice through oxidation.

Generally, two types of juice extractors (juicers) may be considered. Centrifugal juicers function by introducing the food into the open center of the juicer, where the material passes against a rotating metal blade crushing fruits and vegetables into pulp and juice. The pulp is separated from the juice by a using a centrifugal force to propel the juice through a fine mesh filter. The high throughput centrifugal juicer does introduce oxygen and heat, leading to somewhat diminished raw nutrient content. Unfortunately, the extremely high relative rpm (3000-14,0000) kill many of the enzymes offered by fresh juices. Generally, the less expensive or older the centrifugal juicer is, the higher the potential for oxidation during processing. The good news is that many fast-processing centrifugal juicers are operating at slower rpms or have other mechanisms in place to address excess, harmful heat. And the prices of such juicers continue to fall. For example, the dutiful Breville is equipped with a mechanism to "dial in" the relative hardness or softness of fruits and vegetables and the speed of the rotating blade is adjusted accordingly.

For those interested in harvesting the maximum amount of nutritional value, a masticating or cold juicer is recommended to avoid excessive breakdown and oxidation of the ingredients during processing. A masticating juicer features a slowly-rotating, central gear-driven auger designed to crush the contents introduced through the vertical orifice. The juice flows by gravimetric action through a downward oriented channel into a collection vessel, while the pulp is collected separately. The low rpm range ensures that the vital live enzymes and nutrients remain active once they reach your glass.

Triturating twin gear juicers provide the highest assurance of low oxidation and extracting the most nutrients – for a significant price. Twin gear juicers operate by pressing matter through two, tightly interconnected gears. The pressing action of these gears literally rolls the juice from the pulp, thereby extracting the maximum amount of yield per volume. Operating at the very low end of the rpm spectrum, triturating juicers avoid the damaging oxidation effect of high residual heat from blade friction or introduction of air. It is said that twin gear juicers can be less effective at juicing citrus fruits and can be difficult to clean all the parts.

Finally, the frequency of use and intended juicing volume will play a key role in your selection. Some juicers are equipped with a pulp extractor allowing continually juicing without having to pause to empty the pulp collector. Other aspects include the relative quietness and speed, durability. Naturally, the desired functionality must be balanced against the price range – and the range is considerable. If you are willing to be a bit more creative, second hand juicers abound on Craigslist and other outlets for resale goods. Many receive juicers as a gift or purchase them with the best of intentions, only to find their enthusiasm rapidly wane. On page two of my Chicago-based Craigslist search, I've just located an Omega Vert (shown below) for $160 compared to the list price of around $375.

Table 4: Comparative Summary of Juicer Types

Parameter	Juicer Type		
	Centrifugal	Masticating	Twin-gear Triturating
Good for citrus?	yes	yes	yes
Good for vegetables with stems?	no	yes	yes
Good for nuts?	no	yes	yes
Good for leafy greens?	no	yes	yes
Can process wheatgrass?	no	yes	yes
Relative noise	loud	quiet	quiet
Relative speed	fast	slow	slowest
Revolutions per minute (rpms)	high	low	lowest
Pulp Removal	manual or automatic	manual or automatic	automatic
Clean-up	More difficult	Less difficult	More difficult

Heat generation	high	low	lowest
Relative price	$150 -300	$250 - 400	$500 -1000

Figure 3: Breville® Juicer Fountain™ Plus (Centrifugal Juicer)

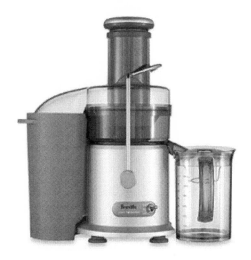

Figure 4: Omega VRT350 Juicer (Masticating Juicer)

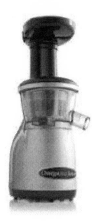

Figure 5: Omega Twin Gear Juicer TWN30S

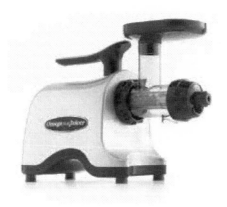

What can't be juiced?

Before you are turned loose in the kitchen with your juicer, perhaps a word of caution is in order. There are some foods which do not lend themselves to juicing either because of their consistency, lack of water content or the presence of toxic compounds, which can accumulate in the processed juice. That said, the list is very short, which further supports the argument that fruit, and vegetables were meant to be consumed in large quantities for good health.

Soft-Fruits-Bananas, Avocados, Mangos

> Soft fruits and vegetables, such as avocados, bananas and mangos generally do not juice well and are best processed in a blender.

Citrus Peel

While a bit of citrus peel provides a healthy dose of limonene, a wonderfully beneficial natural oil associated with digestive and reflux, anti-oxidant and detoxification properties, the human body is not equipped to digest the oils of citrus peels from grapefruit and oranges. Lemons and limes are fine in small doses, but I still tend to juice no more than half a lemon peel for a single serving.

Carrot Tops

There is some debate about whether carrot tops are actually poisonous. I have personally avoided them and substituted other greens into my juices. Carrot roots pose absolutely no threat.

Nightshade Family

Eggplant and tomato belong to the nightshade family, a relatively large genus which contains several highly poisonous members. Eggplant contains solanine, which is even more concentrated in the leaves of tomato plants. To prevent potential concentration of the poisonous alkaloid, the eggplant or tomato leaves should be avoided (tomato fruit is healthy, delicious and free of harmful toxins, however).

Rhubarb Leaves

Rhubarb leaves contain oxalic acid- a compound which accumulates in the kidney and can lead to kidney failure if consumed in high doses. While the amount required to lead to sickness is high, it is wiser to avoid the risk altogether given the myriad combinations of healthy juices and smoothies available.

Wild Parsnips

This book does not contain parsnip recipes but be aware that wild parsnips contain several highly poisonous compounds.

Order of Operations

Does the order in which ingredients are added matter for juicing? Because the flavor of the juice is a combination of the ingredients which are added successively, I find no difference in the taste of the juice by varying the order. There is, however, a practical consideration behind the order when using a masticating juicer (one that grinds produce). I recommend introducing first the leafy greens, then the ingredients which tend to break into tiny bits (e.g. carrots, sweet potato, beets) and chasing these with the more fibrous produce, such as celery, pears or apples. This method allows the fiber to push out the messy bits and renders the screen and base far easier to clean.

Juice Fasts

A juice fast is a type of temporary detoxification diet in which juice is consumed in place of solid foods. Of course, in keeping with the theme of this book, only fresh, unpasteurized, natural juices are permitted as part of juice fasting.[1] Much controversy surrounds the

---

[1] *Quick Tip: Because they do not contain preservatives, fresh juices will spoil*

phenomenon of juice fasting and our aim is to arm the reader with some information to make his or her own decision about whether this program should be pursued. Call it a fad or miracle cure, the juice fast has received an enormous amount of attention thanks to Hollywood stars, nutritionist-bloggers and juice proponents.

The duration and routine of the fast have countless variations, but all rely on the use of liquids to promote a detoxification step over some period. The prevailing thought is that a juice diet provides essential vitamins, minerals, enzymes all the while allowing the digestive system to "rest". Because the body is not taxed with digestion, it can turn its attention to healing and detoxification. Additionally, the high fluid content provides a means to flush released toxins from the body. Purported benefits range from increased energy and focus, weight loss, boosting the immune system, improving skin condition and complexion. We will consider some of the arguments for and against juice fasting.

Typical juice fasts for beginners are 3-4 days in length. Irrespective of the length of the fast, a "bookend" approach is usually employed in which raw foods, fruits and vegetables are consumed prior to, and following, the fast to smooth the transition from whole foods to juices. Additionally, the faster should avoid introduction of any toxins before and after the fast, including, caffeine, nicotine, meat-based proteins and alcohol. It has been reported that serious damage may result from failure to observe

---

more quickly than store bought juices from oxygen from the air. Juice sealers provide an excellent way to store juices in the refrigerator for up to about a week. I have had good success with Vacufresh® brand storage containers.

this. The further away one resides from an all-natural or all-raw foods diet, the more difficult the adjustment expected.

Proponents Argue

Well-known nutritionist and juice pioneer Cherie Calbom recommends a juice cleanse at least twice a year to counter the accumulation of environmental toxins our body is exposed to. She posits that "substances that are not broken down and excreted are generally stored in the intestines, gallbladder, kidneys, liver, fat cells and skin." The claims seem almost fantastic: loss of wrinkles, improved skin coloring, differences in hair and nails texture, increased vitality and energy.

Juices "rest" the major organs involved in digestion and detoxification, giving your stomach, gut and liver a much-earned rest and opportunity to repair. The immune system then can take charge and begin to clear out the dead and damaged cells accumulating in the organs. Calbom recommends juice, rather than water alone, to ensure that the toxins expelled from the cells are bound by the minerals and nutrients in the juices to facilitate their release. A note of caution applies to those who suffer from diabetes or hypoglycemia. Consumption of fruit juices should be avoided and high starch juices like beet and carrot should be diluted sufficiently with an equal amount of water to avoid rapid sugar uptake. Juice fasts promote weight loss. While juice fasts are not meant to be permanent, a minimum 3-day fast can provide the activation to begin a diet.

Joe Cross, author of bestseller, *The Reboot with Joe Juice Diet*, and *Fat, Sick and Nearly Dead*, sustained himself on plant-based juices for

©2018 Kevin Finn

sixty days and then transitioned to a solid plant-based diet for the subsequent three months[15]. In total, Joe Cross maintained the five-month period on the plant-based diet and likened it a "kind of circuit breaker to reset (his) food habits". Cross argues that our bodies were naturally built for detoxification. Consider our organs - kidneys, lymphatic systems, bowels, liver – all play a vital role in detoxifying the body. The combination of increasing levels of xenobiotics (foreign chemicals), poor diets, prescription drugs, alcohol and little exercise contribute to dramatically hinder the efficiency of the natural detoxification systems. A juice "Reboot" is the opportunity to reset the body back into balance by consuming a plant-only juice diet for a defined period. Joe Cross offers various structured juice programs in the book and on his website, https://www.rebootwithjoe.com.

Cross's juice categorizes his juices by color (e.g. red, yellow, green, purple or orange) and each characteristic color is derived from a principal vegetable or fruit. Green juices contain leafy greens, red juices typically include beets, for instance. Rotation among this "palette" of color juices ensures consumption of a more varied spectrum of vitamins and minerals. Joe's juice program spans from a minimum three-day cleanse to a ten-day juice detox regimen. A representative three-day program which Joe presented on Dr. Oz's program is outlined in **Table 5**.[16]

Table 5: Representative 3-day Juice Cleanse Developed by Joe Cross

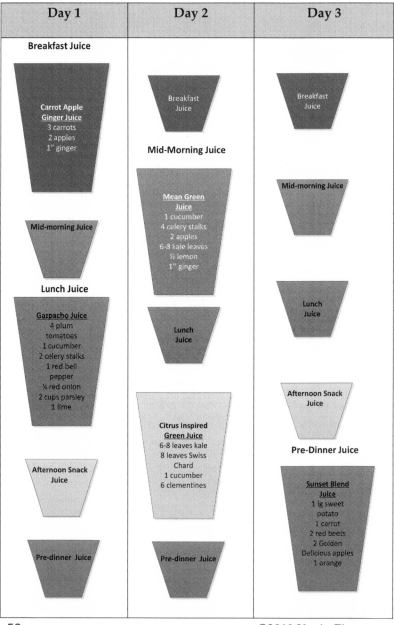

Day 1	Day 2	Day 3

Breakfast Juice

Carrot Apple Ginger Juice
3 carrots
2 apples
1" ginger

Breakfast Juice

Breakfast Juice

Mid-Morning Juice

Mid-morning Juice

Mean Green Juice
1 cucumber
4 celery stalks
2 apples
6-8 kale leaves
½ lemon
1" ginger

Mid-morning Juice

Lunch Juice

Gazpacho Juice
4 plum tomatoes
1 cucumber
2 celery stalks
1 red bell pepper
¼ red onion
2 cups parsley
1 lime

Lunch Juice

Lunch Juice

Afternoon Snack Juice

Citrus Inspired Green Juice
6-8 leaves kale
8 leaves Swiss Chard
1 cucumber
6 clementines

Afternoon Snack Juice

Pre-Dinner Juice

Afternoon Snack Juice

Pre-dinner Juice

Pre-dinner Juice

Sunset Blend Juice
1 lg sweet potato
1 carrot
2 red beets
2 Golden Delicious apples
1 orange

Opponents argue

While they can be a good way to press the "restart button," it isn't scientifically proven that your body needs to be cleansed. "Your body is pretty high tech, and if you think about it, it cleanses itself pretty frequently," says Leslie Schilling, R.D., Memphis-based nutrition counselor.

A day or two is likely safe, she says, but if you're on a cleanse for an extended period of time, you could end up hypocaloric, and your body is going to start tapping into fat stores, forcing the liver to releasing glucose and eventually breaking down muscle tissue. The lack of protein in the juice diet is another consideration. Muscle and connective tissue maintenance requires a steady intake of protein, which pure "juice only" diets lack.

"It really depends on the person and how much extra storage they have lying around," says Schilling. "But within three or four days you're going to see somebody potentially tap into other stores once their body realizes it's not getting the energy it needs from sources like fat and protein." Temporary weight loss is the natural result of a diet without protein and drastically reduced calories. The body has natural mechanisms to detoxify (e.g. liver enzymes). Again, it is difficult to determine whether the juice is *detoxifying* the body

In Verne Varona's *Nature's Cancer Fighting Foods*, we learn that the average life span of red blood cells is approximately four months[17]. Varona indicates that it is our diet over the last four months which dictates our blood chemistry and that, only as blood chemistry changes through the foods we eat, nourishment and healing in other parts of the body may follow in due course. The progression follows from red blood cells to muscle cells, organs nerve and bone such that in approximately seven years' time a complete cellular renewal process occurs. This gradual process of regeneration would then seem at odds with a "quick miracle" detox. Such a detox regime would be expected to cleanse a portion of the body, but a longer period requires for long-term foundational changes in health.

Before embarking on a juice-cleanse, make sure you're cleared with your personal physician and in good health – sound practice when considering any new diet. Cherie Calbom, M.S., author of numerous "Juice Lady" volumes, recommends that those with hypoglycemia will avoid sweet fruit juices and consider diluting carrot juice with equal parts water. Diabetics should be cleared by a doctor and children under 18 should not embark on a fast unless under a physician's care.[18] Most juice fast proponents recommend resting your entire body during this reset period; continuing a rigorous exercise program may deprive you of much needed calories. The juicing endeavor may be an important milestone and learning experience on the path to better health. Changing human behavior is a tough proposition. Such a 3-day juice jolt might be just the thing someone needs to break into or break out of an existing diet or lifestyle habit and set a new course toward a healthier lifestyle.

Chemical, Mineral and Nutrient Components-An Introduction

Antioxidants

The human body is an exquisitely complex machinery involving thousands of chemical reactions occurring with great specificity and selectivity. A great number of these reactions occur through the intermediacy of molecular oxygen, a compound representing approximately 20% of the air we breathe. Somewhat surprisingly, oxygen is the principle compound within group of molecules called reactive oxygen species (ROS). Each of these species has a chemical structure in which an electron is unpaired, rending it more unstable and prone to reaction to achieve a more stable state. The unpaired electron is termed a *"free radical."* Free radical reactions are central to several biological processes; however, uncontrolled free radical reactions can be harmful. If unchecked, oxygen free radicals will seek reactive partners in DNA, proteins and lipids. Quite intuitively, we can imagine that we would not want our DNA and proteins to be compromised through reaction. In fact, we know that replication (copying) of aberrant DNA causes genetic mutation and damage to vital proteins, hampering their ability to properly function and results in disturbances to cellular processes. The origin of many cancers lies in damaged DNA. Free radical oxidative damage is also associated with UV radiation from the sun's rays and environmental exposures such as chemicals and smoke. Fortunately, the human body has a variety of mechanisms to ensure that free radical reactive species are held in check and do not run rampant, causing uncontrolled cellular damage. As their name implies, antioxidants serve as a regulator of the reactive oxidant species. They perform this function by trapping dangerous free radicals before they react with DNA or other vital compounds. Antioxidants are found in all living things. The beauty is that, humans can ingest antioxidants from the plant kingdom and enjoy enhanced protection from plant-based antioxidants. The *same antioxidants* concentrated in the skins of fruits to protect them from free radicals caused by the sun's radiation exert the same protective effects when we eat these foods. Super antioxidants include vitamin C (ascorbic acid), vitamin E, beta-carotene, ellagic acid, betalains, reverstrol, flavonoids.

Carotenoids

Carotenoids refer to class of more than 600 richly colored pigments produced by plants. They are a kind of natural "solar collector", evolutionarily adapted to absorb the maximum amount of light at the correct wavelength along the electromagnetic spectrum to optimize photosynthesis, the process through which plants absorb carbon dioxide, water and sunlight to make their own food. The powerful carotenoid solar harvesters play a dual role as plant antioxidants. As it turns out, carotenoids impart their antioxidant properties to us when we ingest them. Commonly encountered carotenoids include beta-carotene, which is responsible for the color of carrots, and lycopene, which gives tomatoes their characteristic hue. Beta-carotene, along with alpha-carotene and beta-cryptoxanthin are converted in the body to provitamin A.[19] The National Institutes of Health characterizes vitamin A as a group of fat-soluble retinoids, among them retinol, retinal and retinyl esters. As their name suggests, these provitamin A derivatives are associated with the retinal receptors in the eye and thus required for proper vision. Carotenoid champions include tomato juice, carrots, spinach, broccoli and sweet potatoes.

Chlorophyll

Chlorophyll is molecule central to the photosynthetic process, the mechanism by which plants convert carbon dioxide and light energy to water, oxygen and energy. It is this process which generates the sugars which serve as a food source. The amazingly complex pathway from light-harvesting of plants to release of oxygen and water begins with capture of the sun's rays from chlorophyll. Perhaps more remarkable is the striking structural similarity between chlorophyll and the hemoglobin molecule in the common porphyrin ring system. Chlorophyll is unique to the plant world (and cyanobacteria), but its related heme group is an important constituent of the hemoglobin protein, the oxygen carrier in our red blood cells. The similarity is shown in **Figure 6**.

Figure 6: Structural Similarity between Chlorophyll and Hemoglobin[20]

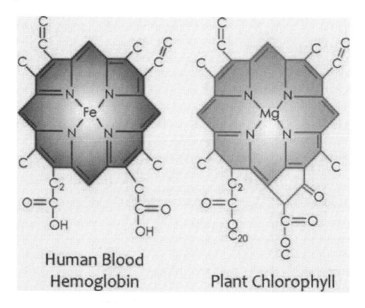

Human Blood Hemoglobin   Plant Chlorophyll

It turns out that ingestion of chlorophyll improves blood function, possibly through conversion of the chlorophyll molecule to the all-important heme group found in the hemoglobin making up our red blood cells. While links to chlorophyll consumption and red blood cell function are known, the exact mechanism is yet to be elucidated. Improvement in red blood cell function has far-reaching benefits[21], including increased energy, combating anemia and prevention of carbon dioxide accumulation in the blood. Chlorophyll is an antioxidant and has been demonstrated to bind toxins to facilitate their clearance from the body.[22] Natural chlorophyll is obtained from spinach, kale, cereal grasses (such as wheat, oats, barley), broccoli, bell peppers, Swiss chard, seaweed, algae, etc.

Enzymes

From building muscle to cell signaling, enzymes lie at the center of all vital biochemical processes. Enzymes are (almost always) proteins specially adapted to facilitate biochemical reactions through their 3-dimensional structure. One of the classes of protein enzymes to be well characterized is the protease, an enzyme which, ironically aids in the digestion of proteins. The enzymatic digestion process is one of the first events in the breakdown of foods to release nutrients for nourishment of the body. Proteases are also found outside the animal kingdom. Fruits also contain enzymes like proteases those naturally secreted during digestion. Among these, *bromelain* from pineapple and *papain* in papaya are particularly well studied. Juicing allows the intact enzyme to be ingested, conferring in the case of bromelain and papain, the digestive properties from the enzyme. Processed or store-bought juices are often pasteurized which render the enzymes inactive.

Fats and Fatty Acids

Unsaturated fats, trans-fats, monounsaturated fats and polyunsaturated fats comprise the four classes of dietary fats. Unsaturated fats are those typically present in animal products, especially red meat and are associated with elevated cholesterol, heart disease and obesity. These fats form the basis of the stereotypical "fatty" diet. Trans- fats are unnatural chemical compounds developed as an alternative to saturated fats and these should also be avoided. Olive oil is a monounsaturated fat and has been linked to raising LDL (good cholesterol), lowering HDL (bad cholesterol) and reducing the risk of heart disease.

Polyunsaturated fatty acids include the Essential Fatty Acids (EFAs) omega-3-linoleic and omega-6-linoleic acids. The term "essential" in the nutritional context refers to those which cannot be made in the body and must be ingested from external sources. They are, in fact, essential in that we require them to sustain life. The ratio of omega-6- to omega-3 fatty acids is an important determinant of health.[23] Omega-6 fatty acids are available from grains and vegetable oils and are ubiquitous in the Western diet. It has been suggested that the optimum ratio of omega-6-fatty acids to omega-3-fatty acids is about 2:1. The modern North American diet has tipped this balance closer to 20:1 or even 30:1. The balance can be restored by introducing a higher proportion of protective omega-3s into our diets. These fatty acids are found in fish oils, leafy greens, rapeseed oil and flax seed. Omega-3's are also key building blocks of the brain and are implicated in cell signaling and brain function. Inflammatory response, depression and fetal development in pregnant mothers are also linked to omega-3 levels.[24] The tendency of omega-3 fatty acids to thin blood makes them a natural heart helper. Omega-3-friendly foods include Avocados, pumpkin seeds, flax seeds, spinach.

Fiber

Dietary fiber is simply the bulk of material from the foods we eat that cannot be absorbed or digested. Found in fruit, vegetables, legumes and grains, fiber plays an extensive role in maintaining good health. Fiber is further classified as "insoluble" or "soluble". Insoluble fiber is found in potatoes, whole grains, celery, carrots, root vegetables, wheat bran, nuts and beans. This is the sort that helps move material through the digestive system and is therefore associated with good colon health.

Soluble fiber also plays an important role as a regulator of blood sugar and reducer of LDL (bad) cholesterol. Soluble fiber is found in apples, cucumbers, oranges, bananas, pears, blueberries and oatmeal.[25] According to a recent Mayo Clinic Staff article, soluble fiber acts to diminish the rate of the sugar absorption and help improve blood sugar levels. They conclude that a "healthy diet that includes insoluble fiber may also reduce the risk of developing type 2 diabetes."[26] Finally, on a per volume basis, high fiber foods tend to be less dense and therefore constitute an integral part of a weight maintenance or weight loss regimen. The market for fiber supplements is an enormous business. Should you take supplements to meet the American Dietetic Association's daily recommended requirements of 21-38 g of fiber? Joanne Lupton, a spokesperson for the American Society of Nutrition and professor of nutrition at Texas A&M University says: "The real issue here is that eating a high-fiber diet from foods is almost, by definition, an excellent diet," said "It's hard to reach dietary fiber recommendations without eating a lot of fiber … so once you take it out of the food, you probably won't have a very good diet."[27] The smoothies found in this book provide a great start toward achieving the recommended daily amount of fiber.

Magnesium

The distribution of magnesium is principally split between 60% in the skeleton and 27% in the muscle; only about 6-7% is found in various cells or external to the cell.[28] Magnesium plays a central role in catalyzing hundreds of enzymatic reactions, from protein synthesis to conversion of fats and carbohydrates to energy to cell signaling and ion transport processes. Because of its critical function in such varied metabolic processes, deficiency of magnesium has disastrous consequences such as improper Ca regulation, imbalance of sodium and potassium, nerve and muscular impairment and gastroenteric issues. Deficiency is rare in healthy adults because of the wide distribution of magnesium in many foods but can be observed in alcoholics and those with renal disorders. Magnesium is abundantly found in spinach, celery, carrots, beets and broccoli. Smoothie additives, like almonds, tofu and avocado are also great sources of magnesium.

Polysaccharides

Our main source of energy is fuel from carbohydrates. A relatively new diet craze has wrongly implicated carbohydrates as dietary "bad guys". The truth, however, is that *carbohydrate (or sugar)* is a generic term for a class of organic molecules composed of carbon, hydrogen and oxygen. Simple carbohydrate such as fructose and glucose are monosaccharides- single units of sugar. It is this class of *simple sugar carbohydrates* which pose concern for dietary health. Simple sugars are found in processed breads, chips, sweets and candies and can contribute to diabetes if consumed in excess and over long periods of time. In contrast, *complex carbohydrates* are represented by polysaccharides, a group of molecules composed of repeating units of glucose which are generally slower to be digested by human enzymes. It is especially the low glycemic polysaccharides such as those found in sweet potatoes, whole grain pasta and fruits which require a longer time for digestion, steadying blood sugar contributing to better health. New research also highlights the various nutritional roles of non-starch polysaccharides, a carbohydrate found in plant cell walls.[29] Pectins, cellulose correspond to dietary fiber and demonstrate the same properties of insoluble and soluble fiber, namely nutritional benefits of colon and digestive system and lowering of blood sugar and cholesterol levels, respectively.

Phytonutrients

Rooted in *"phyto"*, the Greek word for plant, a phytonutrient refers to a member of the more than 25,000 chemical compounds of plant origin. Phytonutrients are organic molecules evolutionarily adopted into a plant's biological processes to assist in its survival; these diverse functions may include protection from insects, chemical metabolites, photosynthesis/ light harvesting, and antioxidant protection. The term phytochemical is preferred by some experts to differentiate it from nutrients in the true sense, which are those chemicals entities required to sustain life. Examples of phytonutrients include carotenoids, flavonoids, ellagic acid and polyphenols, and phytoestrogen.

Phytoestrogens

Phytoestrogens, a class of compounds similar in chemical structure to the natural estrogen molecule, are thought to be produced by plants as a defense mechanism[30]. The prevailing theory is that, ingestion of phytoestrogens by herbivores (plant-eating animals) interferes with their fertility, thereby limiting the number of offspring (natural predators) of the plant. Introducing such "infertility" chemicals in the food source is a plant's way of starving out, and therefore; staving off, its pool of predators.

Phytoestrogens resemble the natural steroid estrogen in its shape and molecular properties and, as such, acts as a mimic of estrogen by binding to estrogen receptors[31]. Phytoestrogens naturally occur in soy products- a central component of the typical Asian diet. The lower prevalence of certain cancers among Asian populations spurred the investigation of the relationship between soy products and cancer. As higher levels of blood estrogen often correlate to elevated risk of breast cancer, the presence of phytoestrogen may attenuate the production of natural estrogen, though other mechanisms are possible, including influence of protein synthesis, cell metabolism, enzymes, etc.[32] Other potential benefits include lowering cholesterol, combating osteoporosis and modulating hormones, which can reduce the negative effects of menopause. Again, we find that it is difficult to disentangle the potential effects from phytoestrogen from those benefits garnered through a mainly plant-based diet. We do know that phytoestrogens contain a powerful antioxidant effect which offers protection from various diseases, regardless the mechanism. Of the foods featured in this book, flaxseed contains the highest number of phytoestrogens and possesses beneficial dietary fibers, both insoluble and soluble[33]. Dried fruits, such as dates, peaches and apricots have concentrated levels of phytoestrogens. Strawberries, blueberries and raspberries contain lower amounts.

Proteins

Proteins are large molecules composed of various combinations of amino acids. The nature and function of proteins is determined by the sequence and composition of its constituent amino acid building blocks. Proteins are required for building and maintaining muscle, hair, bones and skin. They also serve as catalysts in biochemical reactions and participate in nearly every cellular process. Because proteins have a finite lifespan, they must be regenerated throughout the lifetime of the organism. To obtain the requisite building blocks to fuel the synthesis of new proteins, we must ingest proteins from food sources. These food-derived proteins are broken down through digestion to amino acid building blocks and re-synthesized into proteins to fuel new cellular processes. How are proteins synthesized from amino acids? With the help of other proteins! Though most associate proteins with animal sources, proteins are present in animal and plants. Meat proteins are termed "complete proteins" because they contain all the nine requisite amino acids to build all the proteins we require. That is, of the twenty amino acids required to build human protein, nine of them must be introduced through the foods we consume. Though plant proteins from single sources are "incomplete", eating a plant and legume diet provides complementary sourcing of amino acids to supply the necessary building blocks for protein synthesis. It is very easy for vegetarians to consume the full complement of the essential amino acids through pairing foods. For example, rice and beans contain all the necessary amino acids without reliance on meat. Some plant protein powerhouses featured in the book include: avocado, spinach, kale, pumpkin, chia seeds. Tofu is a great source of vegetable protein and lends itself well to smoothies as it takes on the flavor of the other blended components. The addition of tofu to a smoothie is a healthier alternative to "beefing up" smoothies with yogurt or cow's milk.

Vitamin C

Ascorbic acid, commonly called Vitamin C, is a small, water-soluble molecule which humans require from nutritional sources. That is, humans are incapable of producing their own vitamin C. In contrast, most plants and animals can synthesize this vitamin in the organism and do not require its ingestion. Vitamin C is therefore essential to humans and plays several roles as a cofactor in various biochemical reactions. A cofactor is a molecule which assists a protein in a biochemical process and in this context, vitamin C assists in synthesis of biomolecules, such as carnitine and collagen. We have presented it in this context as a powerful antioxidant, where it can preserve DNA and RNA to damage by free radical damage. Several studies have associated vitamin C-through its dietary source-with reduced risk of coronary heart disease, stroke, hypertension (high blood pressure) and a host of cancers.[34] Vitamin C is also vital for maintenance of good immune health. The juices and smoothies throughout this book claimed to combat colds feature many citrus fruits high in vitamin C.

Vitamin K

Vitamin K has been receiving increased attention in the last years; however, the discovery of this fat-soluble compound dates to 1929. The "K" is derived from the German word of blood clotting (*Koagulation*) because of its principal role in connection with blood clotting phenomenon. Vitamin K is associated with electron capture in photosynthetic plants and therefore is found in high abundance in green, leafy vegetables. Its intake has been connected to reduced risk of osteoporosis, cancer, heart disease and Type II diabetes. Kale, spinach, collard greens, parsley represent some of the Vitamin K powerhouses.

Juicing Ingredients and Description

Aloe Vera

Aloe has been employed in a wide range of medicinal and cosmetic applications for over 5,000 years. Though the aloe plant resembles a cactus in its spiny, tapered green leaves, aloe belongs to the tree lily family. Of the more than 250 varieties of aloe, *Aloe barbadensis* is the most common commercially grown variety. According to WebMD, aloe plants produce two medically useful components: the gel and the latex. Aloe gel is the clear, gelatinous substance found in the inner plant leaf. The healing sap of the aloe plant is widely used in cosmetics and skin products to strengthen hair and nail and provides effective natural remedy for burns and sunburn. Additionally, the yellow bitter part of the aloe can be orally ingested as a laxative. Aloe provides treatment against bowel diseases including ulcerative colitis and stomach ulcers; it is a natural intestinal cleanser and is associated with reduction of digestive inflammation. The antioxidative and detoxifying action provide relief of some side effects of radiation treatment.[57] Aloe gel is bitter to the taste and is best rendered into a smoothie with sweet fruits such as pineapple, mango or berries to balance the tartness.

Apples

The over 7,500 varieties of apples are members of the rose family. Apples provide an excellent source of natural fiber and vital minerals. The compound quercetin, found in red apples, has been implicated in stimulation of the immune system. Studies[35] have demonstrated a scientific link between consumption of apples and lowering of cholesterol. Dr. Bahram H. Arjmandi, PhD, RD, of Florida State University, conducted a study in which 160 women of two study groups were directed to eat either dried apples or dried prunes for a year. Not only did the study group associated with apple consumption demonstrate a marked 23% decrease in LDL (bad cholesterol) after 6 months, this group experienced weight loss on the average of 3.3 lbs. Apples are great for juicing because they provide a good yield and delicious sweetness to balance acidity or tartness. It is reported that over half of the vitamin C content is found near the surface of the skin; for maximizing the health benefit, the entire apples except the core should be consumed.[36]

Avocado

Carotenoids and vitamin E antioxidants found in avocados are vital for protection against damaging oxidation from chemicals, aging and the sun's rays. The omega-3 and oleic fatty acids maintain essential hydration of the lipids in the epidermal layer. Avocados are rich in phytosterols, which inhibit the absorption of cholesterol and thereby lower the amount of LDL (bad cholesterol). The same phytosterols are associated with anti-inflammatory activity. High in vitamin K, pantothenic acid, copper, potassium, folate and avocados are among the most healthful foods[36]. Adding an avocado to a smoothie is a great way to make it more filling. The exterior skin of an avocado should be dark brown and yield slightly to the touch while the center should be mostly green. Brown meat is a sign of overripe or damaged avocado. For easy peeling, cut lengthwise around the entire fruit and pull in half. To remove the pit, tap a sharp knife into center of pit and turn one quarter turn to free. Scoop out contents with a spoon.

Banana

Did you know that the banana belongs to the same family as the lily and the orchid? It is said that the word "banana" is derived from the Arabic word for finger (*banan*), and, as such, the early Arabic slave traders are given credit for the name.[36] Bananas provide potassium, vitamin B6, vitamin C, fiber and well as a slow-digesting source of carbohydrates, which prevents spike in blood sugar[36, 37]. The importance of potassium cannot be overstated. Potassium acts as a natural substitute for sodium and thereby lowers the sodium level in the body. When sodium levels are high, the body retains water to restore the balance of sodium in the cells. It is likely that excesses of sodium lead to slightly expanded blood volume, a phenomenon that may, in turn, increase blood pressure. A higher intake of potassium can reverse this cascade of events, lowering blood pressure and reducing the risk of heart problems. Bananas[2] add creaminess and sweetness to smoothies, but do not lend themselves to juicing because of their low water content. They may also be cut and frozen for months.

---

[2] *Quick Tip: Bananas can be frozen for approximately two months. To reduce degrative effects of oxidation, treat with a little lemon juice prior to storage.*

Beet

The leaves (greens)[3] and tubers of beets[4] are edible and extremely nutritious. Beets come in several varieties: purple, red, yellow and belong to the same family as spinach, chard and kale. Red or purple coloring denotes high betalain content whereas vulgaxanthin gives yellow beets their characteristic color. Both species offer protective antioxidant properties which are enjoyed in cooked and juiced beets. Beets serve as a cleanser for the liver, possess aphrodisiac properties and are a rich source of powerful antioxidants, such as betalain and b-carotene. They are a low-calorie energy source and are high in vitamin A and nearly every metabolically essential mineral[38] such as iron, calcium, manganese, potassium and magnesium.[39] Beets are a natural source of nitrates, triggering a chain of nitric oxide synthase to open blood vessels and increase blood flow. Increased blood flow may alleviate symptoms of cardiovascular disease, reduce inflammation and increase blood flow to provide a welcome "rise" to certain extremities. To prepare: Peel the hard, outer skin to expose the brightly colored meat. Because of their fibrous root, they are best processed using a juicer. The leaves should be cleaned by washing

---

[3] *Quick Tip: Beets only keep 3-4 days in the refrigerator with the roots attached because the leaves require moisture provided by the root. It is best to remove the beet greens prior to storage*

[4] *Quick Tip: Beets and carrots tend to leave a difficult-to-remove residue on the plastic parts of the juicer. I've found this film to be resistant to removal with detergent, water or vinegar. Try dampening a soft cloth with olive oil and rubbing gently to remove this deposit.*

in cold water. Beet greens are an excellent addition to juices and smoothies.[5]

Blackberries

Known to have some of the highest levels of chemo-preventative and antibacterial anthocyanins and ellagic acid among fruits, blackberries are also rich in Vitamin C, folate and manganese[38]. Blackberry seeds contain omega-3 and omega-6 fatty acids, are among the highest berries in calcium and have been shown to reduce risk of kidney stones through action of the proanthocyanin compounds. In North America, they are generally in season May through August, though it is now common to find them frozen in grocery stores. The frozen variety make an easy addition to smoothies year-round but should be used frozen as thawing will render them mushy.

Blueberries

Blueberries-one of the few fruits whose majority of species are native to North America, are another of Dr. Steven Pratt's 14 Superfoods. Though somewhat lower in Vitamin C, these berries more than supplant this property in their high antioxidant content, especially flavonoids (polyphenols), ellagic acid and anthocyanins. Moreover, blueberries have been demonstrated to improve memory function. Their antioxidants contribute toward lowering

---

[5] *Quick Tip: Beet juice stains can be removed from clothing by washing with cold water immediately. For persistent stains, soak a piece of white bread in ice water. Apply directly to stain for several minutes. The stain should be lifted into the bread.*

of blood pressure through action of nitric oxide and those affected with Type II diabetes have been shown to benefit by balancing blood sugar levels. Blueberries should be washed and eaten with the skin on to extract the maximum nutritional content. Fortunately, blueberries can be safely frozen without diminishing their nutritional content.

Cantaloupe

According to a recent article in Medical News Today, cantaloupe provides 106% of the recommended daily value of vitamin A, 95% of the target value of vitamin C, 1% of calcium and 2% of iron needs.[40] The b-carotene and related carotenoids found in cantaloupe offers protection against prostate cancer.[41] Vitamin C provides antioxidant protection and supports the immune system. Because cantaloupes contain mostly water, they are excellent for hydration, which supports good overall health. Cantaloupes can be added to smoothies or juiced directly.

Cherries

Cherries belong to the same family as apricots, peaches and plums and may be further divided into sour and sweet varieties (also known as pie and tart, respectively). Sour cherries are somewhat higher in vitamin A and possess a lower calorie count. Their characteristic colors are derived from the flavonoid compounds, most notably anthocyanins, which provide antioxidant protection. Gout, a disease characterized by painful accumulation of uric acid in the blood and ultimately the joints, may be alleviated by cherries owing to their ability to inhibit xanthine oxidase, a protein responsible for producing uric acid.[37] The powerful mixture of

©2018 Kevin Finn

phytochemicals in cherries is responsible for the anti-inflammatory and cholesterol-lowering properties.[36]   Sweet cherries may be juiced after removal of the pits and the juice diluted with water or another juice to reduce sweetness.

Cactus Pear Fruit (Tuna)

The cactus has long been exploited in folk medicine and the prickly pear tuna (fruit) has been used in everything from water purification to ointments for burns to the base for an alcoholic drink and- ironically enough- a hangover remedy. The vibrant pink colored center of the cactus fruit is a delicacy in Mexico and is often made into jams or simple syrups. The pectin and fiber are attributed to lowering blood sugar levels by diminishing its adsorption into the stomach and intestine.   It is therefore recommended to alleviate the effects of Type II diabetes. Cactus fruits are high in vitamin C and magnesium and are loaded with protective antioxidants like betalain (as found in beets). The anthocyanins found in cactus have been reported to improve immunity through boosting functioning of white blood cells.[38] The hands should be protected when separating the spiky outer layer from the inner fruit. Begin by cutting the hard, circular portion off the top and bottom. Cut once lengthwise down the center of the fruit. Carefully peel back the outer layer to expose the brightly colored, semi-sweet, flesh. The fruit contains seeds which may be eaten. A masticating juicer, however, will allow the separation of the juice from the seeds.

Coconut

Coconut meat is principally composed of medium chain triglycerides, a rich energy source. They are high in manganese. Additionally, the vitamin A precursor and vitamin E components of coconut meat have been shown to reduce LDL (harmful) cholesterol. These compounds display powerful antioxidant properties and serve as protection against oxidative skin and tissue damage. Coconut meat can be converted to coconut milk as a lactose-free milk substitute, eaten raw, or blended into smoothies. It seems caution is warranted if consumed in excess. Coconuts may not be the superfood once thought, because of their high saturated fat content. Some researchers, most notably Harvard Professor Dr. Karin Michels, have recently denounced coconut oil and instead suggested use of unsaturated fats as a safer alternative.

Coconut Water

Coconut water refers to the sweet, nutty liquid found at the center of a young coconut. Recently, coconut water has enjoyed widespread marketing as "mother nature's sports drink", writes Kathleen M. Zelman, MPH, RD, LD, in an article for WebMD, "The Truth About Coconut Water". Celebrities and marketers have propelled coconut water into the spotlight as a cure for hangovers, kidney stones and even cancer. Coconut water contains less sugar, more potassium and less sodium than most sports drinks and therefore may be better at replacing fluids lost during intense exercise sessions. The bottom line is that coconut water provides a low calorie and perhaps less nauseating means to replace fluids lost during intense exercise. Coconut water – whether fresh or boxed – appears in various smoothie recipe for a little added "potassium" kick.

Grapes

Grapes are among the leading crops in the world and have been cultivated as far back as 5000 B.C. The many antioxidant benefits having been recently associated with wine are also available from their natural sources. Their nutritional benefits are like other berries, having in common phenolic antioxidants such as anthocyanins, resveratrol, phenolic acids and flavonoids.[42] Grapes are rich in mineral content, especially potassium. Researchers at the University of Michigan have demonstrated the benefits of table grapes in protecting the heart, presumably through activation of the antioxidant glutathione, a molecule found in heart cells and known to protect against oxidative stress.[43]

Grapefruit

Besides offering high vitamin C and minerals, the grapefruit is known to have benefits associated with improved red blood cell function. The rind is particularly high in limonene and antioxidants. The salicylic acid in grapefruit is suggested to dissolve calcium deposits resulting in alleviation of arthritis symptoms. The combination of vitamin C, antioxidants and salicylic acid – which loosens mucous – is an ideal natural cold combatant.

To juice, cut into quarters; peel off rind and introduce to juicer. **Warning: if you are taking medication, consult your prescribing physician before eating grapefruit.** These fruits are potent inhibitors of cytochrome 450 oxidases, enzymes responsible for first pass clearance of drugs. Formulation and dosing of drugs is based on normal functioning of metabolizing enzymes such as cytochrome P450 oxidase. Interference with P450s through ingestion of grapefruit may result in an accidental overdose of medication. This warning also applies to starfruit (see below). The pith contains high amounts of limonene. Leave much of this intact to maximize healthful benefits.

Guava

Guavas are Asian fruits which seem to be popping up in Western grocery stores are these health benefits are recognized alongside their deliciously refreshing flavor. Two varieties, the green "apple guava" and the smaller "strawberry guava" are most easily found in Western or Asian food stores in North America. Guavas have no pit and the entire fruit, including seeds and skin, can be eaten (although the dark knotty top portion is best removed). They provide high fiber, vitamin C and niacin,[51] impart a fruity taste, are low in sugar and therefore great for those watching their weight. Additionally, they contain high amounts of lycopene and other antioxidants, are packed with vitamin C and are shown to be beneficial for maintaining younger-looking skin. Finally, they are an astringent and promote teeth and gum health.

Lemons

Like all citrus fruits, lemons are high in vitamin C and contain a host of powerful bioflavonoids which provide cholesterol lowering effects and antioxidant protection. The acidity in lemons renders them natural antiseptic and is a chief component of many home remedies for colds, sore throat, allergies and diarrhea.[51] Lemon juice treatment may also be used to dissolve kidney stones.

Limes

High in vitamin C, limes[6] are great to pair with sweet fruits to lend a sweet and sour flavor. Limes and lemons have digestive enzymes like our own and may help to alleviate bloating and indigestion. Limes are anti-viral and boost the immune system. As with lemons, the highest content of limonene is found in the whitish rind. Limonene is associated with anti-cancer, detoxifying and digestive functions. Limes are most easily juiced by cutting in half and pressing with hand held squeezer. Roll limes on hard surface to increase juiciness.

Lychees

Lychee is a tropical fruit native to southern China having a tough, leathery outer skin covering a deliciously sweet white pulp. It has virtually no saturated fat or cholesterol, but is high in vitamin C, phenolic and flavonoid antioxidants as well as B- vitamins. To access the fruit, cut around the top of the outer shell to expose the white fruit. Gently away the shell and slit the white fruit down to help peel away the fruit from the nut. Discard the nut and outer shell.

---

[6] *Quick Tip: Limes with the thinnest skin are usually the juiciest. These tend to be a bit yellow. For more effective juice extraction, roll the lime back and forth on the countertop using gentle pressure prior to squeezing the lime.*

Kiwis

Kiwis provide high levels of vitamin C, vitamin K, folate and potassium. Additionally, the actindain aids in digestion of proteins. For those having an aversion to bananas, either through allergy or taste, kiwis serve as a great substitute to impart sweetness and creaminess to smoothies. Kiwis do not juice well, however, because of their softness. Ripe kiwis should be firm but yield slightly to the touch. Kiwi fruit is best extracted by cutting the fruit in half and scooping it out with a teaspoon.

Mangos

Mangos have extended beyond their original Indian roots to be found in nearly every grocery store, which is one of the reasons I feature them in so many recipes. Like pineapple, mangos provide a sweetness which balances bitterness of greens and lends a wonderfully fresh and tropical hint to each of the smoothies and juices. They are extremely high in vitamin A and C, demonstrate protection against certain types of cancers.[51] Again, like pineapples, enzymes in mangos are good for aiding in digestion. They are also excellent sources of potassium and niacin.

To prepare: Peel skin with a paring knife or kitchen peeler. Cut in slices, taking care to avoid the bone in the center.

Oranges

The orange is probably the quintessential health food and one of the first to have been recognized for its healthful benefits. Many would be surprised to know that the orange does not provide the highest amount of vitamin C relative to other fruits or even vegetables, such as bell peppers. Despite any disappointment we might associated with its having been dethroned vitamin C champion among fruits, it is one of most healthy foods because of its having vitamin A, folic acid, phosphorous, calcium. The pectin found in the rind is associated with lowering cholesterol.[51] Oranges have remarkable immune-boosting effects and have long been considered a natural cold remedy.

Passion Fruit

Available in yellow and purple varieties, the passion fruit has been shown to possess cytotoxic effects against cancer cells through the power of its polyphenols and carotenoids (among them vitamin A and carotenoid analogues). Several studies connect the anticancer properties specifically to reduction of prostate cancer[38] by lycopene. This carotenoid is also associated with improved vision by protecting the retina. Other uniquely important chemicals include harmala alkaloids, which are structurally and functionally like monooxidase inhibitors used in clinical treatment of depression. Indeed, the passion flower containing higher levels of these alkaloids has been associated with sedative effects. Finally, passion fruit is high in vitamin C and dietary fiber. Selection of the fruit can be performed by first smelling, then shaking the fruit. A ripe passion fruit will smell sweet and aromatic. By comparing the fruits through shaking, you can gauge how densely packed they are with the delicious seeds and juice which you have identified with your nose! Cut the fruit on the outside with a sharp knife and peel back to expose the watery center. Use a spoon to scoop out the contents.

Papayas

Papayas contain high levels of vitamin C, as well as a good mixture of minerals, folate and B-carotene. The protective effects of papayas against colon cancer are attributed to its ability of its fiber to bind to and eliminate toxins as they accumulate in the colon. Vitamin C, vitamin A and the various carotenoids are implicated in stimulating the immune system. Unripe papayas contain higher levels of papain, an enzyme known to combat indigestion, hay fever, chronic diarrhea and trauma.[44]

To ensure proper selection, look for yellowish –green fruits. The skin should be nearly completely yellow when fully ripe.[7] The pressure should be firm but yield slightly to the touch. To expedite ripening, wrap them in newspaper for up to 48 hours before eating. Fruit should be yellowish on the outside when ripe. Peel and discard skin and remove seeds before juicing or addition to smoothies.

Pears

Though pears yield far lower vitamin and mineral content compared to most fruits,[51] the phytonutrient content and insulin-regulating capabilities provide a balanced complement to vegetable and fruit juices. To obtain the maximum benefit of pectin, add them to smoothies rather than juice them. Pears yield a sweet, mild juice which may be used to offset bitterness of vegetable juices. Pears are packed with phenolic antioxidants (especially in the skins). They are loaded with water-soluble fibers

[7] *Quick Tip: To accelerate the ripening of papaya, wrap in newspaper and store at room temperature for 24-48 hours.*

like pectin Pears have been employed as a traditional cough remedy when combined with honey; this recipe has long been used in Asia as a home remedy. In this context, pears can reduce throat irritation and help clear mucous.

Persimmons

According to the California Rare Fruit Growers, persimmons are generally classified into two groups: astringent fruits, that are high in tannins and bear soft fruit when ripe, and non-astringent fruits, which are lower in tannins and remain harder in texture; think of an apple. The former is commonly grown in Japan and are known as "Hachiya". Non-astringent varieties commonly found in the United States include the Fuyu and Gosho. Consistent with their yellow-orange to dark red color, persimmons contain several vitamin A-type carotenoid antioxidants. Additionally, persimmons deliver vitamin C and B-vitamins. Persimmons promote good digestive health and are known to combat gastro-intestinal inflammations[51]. Except for the seed, the entire fruit is edible, and they may be either juiced or added to smoothies for a deliciously sweet flavor.

Pineapple

Pineapple is a favorite among juicers because it is available year-round, provides a tremendous amount of juice per unit volume and balances tartness or bitterness of greens with a deliciously sweet balance. Well known alternative medicine guru Dr. Andrew Weil, M.D. espouses the benefits of pineapples as a natural remedy for trauma healing through the action of bromelain. This adroit enzyme aids in reduction of swelling, acts to digest fibrins from blood clots and is implicated in promoting digestion, alleviating angina, upper respiratory tract infections. Pineapple juice is an effective natural cough suppressant and loosens mucous.[45] Pineapples are high in potassium, which acts as a natural replacement for sodium in the body. Those who eat foods higher in potassium tend to have lower blood pressure through exchange of sodium for potassium.

Pomegranate

Pomegranates[8] contain punicalagin, one of the most powerful antioxidants. This polyphenolic antioxidant bears structural similarity to ellagic acid, which is found in blueberries. This antioxidant seems to be associated with widely beneficial medicinal properties. Pomegranate were shown to clinically reduce blood pressure, reverse formation of atherosclerotic plaques and prevent LDL oxidation as part of a three-year study in which patients were administered pomegranate juice daily.[46]

To prepare pomegranate, cut in two and place halves in ice water for 10 minutes. To separate seeds from the spongy membrane, roll them gently back and forth. Peel membrane to continue exposing the seeds. Perform this under water to avoid splashing the juice. The membrane will float and can be separated from the denser seeds by scooping with a screen filter or pasta scoop.

---

[8] *Quick Tip: Pomegranate has been used as a clothing dye since the times of the ancient Greeks. To help remove pomegranate stains. 1/2 c. milk for hours (even overnight) and then I spot-wash with regular laundry detergent.*

Starfruit

Also called carambola, the starfruit is completely edible. The starfruit boasts high vitamin C content, provides a host of antioxidants and displays antimicrobial activity. **Warning**: because of their relatively high oxalic acid content, they should not be consumed by those suffering from kidney failure or risk of illness or death. **Warning**: if you are taking medication, consult your prescribing physician before eating starfruit. These fruits are potent inhibitors of cytochrome 450 oxidases, enzymes responsible for first pass clearance of drugs. Formulation and dosing of drugs is based on normal functioning of metabolizing enzymes such as cytochrome P450 oxidase. Interference with P450s through ingestion of starfruit may result in an accidental overdose of medication. This warning also applies to grapefruit (see above).

Strawberries

Strawberries are high in vitamin C, manganese, folate and potassium. It is the protective flavonoid antioxidants in the skin which are responsible for imparting the characteristic red color. The flavonoid quercetin, also found in red apples, is known to act as a natural anti-inflammatory agent, alleviating the effects of atherosclerosis. A cup of strawberries provides the same amount of vitamin C as a cup of orange juice and as much fiber as a slice of whole wheat bread.[38]

Raspberries

The antioxidant power derived from anthocyanins and associated with red wines is also available from raspberries. Raspberries are high in vitamin C, potassium, folate. Like most berries, raspberries demonstrate anti-inflammatory effects which have far-reaching health benefits, from weight loss to heart health.

Watermelon

The watermelon has gained notoriety as a lycopene-rich food, an honor which is typically associated with the tomato. Watermelons are abundant in beta carotene, vitamin C and flavonoids. Citrulline, a biochemical precursor to the amino acid arginine is also found in high levels in watermelon. It is thought that the citrulline, once converted to arginine, is responsible for improved blood flow. Cucurbitacin E, an anti-inflammatory compound and cyclooxygenase inhibitor is found in watermelon. The lycopene and B-carotene content of watermelon is highly dependent on its stage of ripeness. Although all parts of watermelon (including the whitish outer rind) contain nutrients, the latest stage of ripeness is associated with higher distribution of lycopene and B-carotene.

Vegetables

Cactus (Nopales)

Nopales are the stems of the cactus plant, a vegetable long-used in the Mexican cuisine as a vegetable. Cactus paddles, in addition to offering vitamins A and C, are rich in non-starch polysaccharides like pectin, mucilage and hemicelluloses. Non-starch polysaccharides lower LDL (bad cholesterol), stabilize blood sugar. Cactus paddles contain phenolic antioxidants at levels approaching berries and are associated with reduced risk of osteoporosis through the action of flavonoid phytochemicals isorhamnetin and kaempferol.[38]

84   ©2018 Kevin Finn

To prepare: wash with cold water to remove dust. With an outward cutting motion, pass a sharp knife parallel with the paddle to remove the sharp spines. Cut away approximately 1/8 around the perimeter to remove the peripheral spines. Cut into strips and blend or juice.

Carrots

Carrots are one of the oldest vegetables, having been cultivated for more than 4,000 years. Their characteristic orange hue is attributed to the high content of the powerful beta-carotene antioxidant. Beta-carotene is the same molecule responsible for maintenance of good vision and protection against macular degeneration. Carrots are associated with reduction in risk of heart disease and various types of cancer.

Celery

Celery provides fiber, appreciable amounts of vitamin C, vitamin K and folate. It provides antioxidant protection owing to polyphenols and flavonoids. Additionally, non-starch polysaccharides, most notably pectin, offer anti-inflammatory benefits. It is a great complement to vegetable juices because of its natural salt. Remove the stalk and wash thoroughly with water. The green leaves may be used as well as the stalk.

Cucumber

Cucumbers are the ultimate food to rejuvenate skin, ligaments and bones. Aside from their power to hydrate, cucumbers are rich in B vitamins, vitamin C, magnesium, folate and polyphenolic antioxidants and silicon. Collagen, a fibrous connective protein tissue which makes up our hair, nails and skin requires silicon. This connective tissue is also essential in maintaining the calcium levels necessary for proper bone regeneration. Certain foods, especially red meat, tend to cause a rise in the acidity level in the body. To buffer this effect and restore the pH balance, calcium may be leached from the bones. Alkaline (basic) foods such as cucumbers can balance the pH and prevent unnecessary erosion of calcium from the bones. Cucumber possess compounds called cucurbitacins which have been implicated in arresting cell signaling processes in cancer pathways, as such, remain important targets in connection with development of anti-cancer drugs. Because they contain up to 95% water, they provide a natural and refreshing source of juice to add pep to your juices. Prepare the cucumber by peeling the outer skin with a peeler or paring knife.

Dandelion Greens

Dandelions are extremely high in b-carotene, potassium, magnesium, folate, b-vitamins and fiber. A true herbal miracle, this weed is a natural liver tonic, treating hepatitis and jaundice, purifies blood through its diuretic capacity[47] and is associated with clear and clean skin. The plant contains high levels of lecithin, a compound which protects against cirrhosis of the liver. The curative effects of dandelion extend to reduction in cholesterol and protection against cancers through action of its antioxidants. Many herbal remedies include dandelions for pain relief and reduction of inflammation. All parts of the plants are edible and may be juiced or added to smoothies. The recipes contained in this book feature the greens, which are purchased organic from the supermarket.

Picking dandelions from the yard should be cautioned, as many grasses in urban and suburban environments contain pesticides.

Fennel

Fennel is composed of edible seeds and a large, aromatic bulb connected to wispy green leaves by a stalk like celery but tasting strongly of aniseed. In fact, fennel belongs to the same vegetable family as carrots, celery and parsley. Its nutritional profile is similar to celery, having vitamin C, folate, and elements like iron and magnesium. Its long-standing use in herbal medicine is derived from four principal actions, as described by Michael Murray, N.D.[44] It is: (1) an intestinal antispasmodic; (2) a carminative agent (one that exerts gas-relieving effects); (3) a compound which strengthens the stomach; (4) an anodyne; a compound which serves as a pain reliever. Fennel has been used in eye batch or as compress to reduce inflammation and as a natural breath freshener! [47] Finally, fennel contains appreciable levels of phytoestrogens, a class of compounds associated with benefits for women. These components include flavonoids rutin, quercitin and kaemferol.[39]

Kale

Despite its green color, kale[9] yields high levels of B-carotene. It is the chlorophyll in the leaves which is responsible for its dark green coloring. A hearty vegetable, kale is packed with Vitamin K, iron

---

[9] *Quick Tip: Spinach and Kale can be processed in a juicer or Vitamix® and frozen in ice cube trays for quick addition of greens to smoothies at a later time.*

and calcium. Kale contains more than twice the levels of antioxidants in most greens making it stand out as a superfood for deterrence of cardiovascular disease and cancers. Its sulforaphane, fiber and high antioxidant content contribute toward its cleansing and detoxifying effects. Sulforaphane is associated with inhibiting bacteria responsible for causing duodenal and stomach ulcers.Error! Bookmark not defined. Kale can be introduced into masticating juicers or blended into smoothies. Red kale has a sweet smell and adds flavor to a smoothie, whereas green kale is more understated (like spinach) and adds bulk and fiber (and a host of vitamins and nutrients) to the smoothie. For smoothies, remove the leafy part from the fibrous center stalk. Kale leaves can be processed whole in juicers, however.

Peppers (Bell, Chili)

Bell peppers belong to the *Capsicum* genus alongside chili peppers; however, the genetic makeup of Bell peppers is marked by a recessive gene which prevents the production of capsaicin, the principal ingredient contributing to spiciness.Error! Bookmark not defined. They are members of the nightshade family which includes tomatoes and eggplant. Aside from providing higher value of vitamin C than an orange, bell peppers contain an astounding array of antioxidants associated with reduction of cancer and cardiovascular diseases. Peppers also represent a great source of folate, vitamin E, B-vitamins and minerals. The intense variation in colors of the peppers is not due to different species, but rather the various states of maturity in which they are harvested. Green bell peppers are harvested prior to full development, while yellow and red peppers are fully mature, lending a milder and -at times-sweeter flavor. The variation in color is caused by differing levels of antioxidants. Red peppers, for instance, contain approximately 10 times the amount of B-carotene than green peppers.

Chili peppers come in many varieties and produce capsaicin in quite varying amounts. These peppers provide an excellent source vitamin C and A; however, care should be taken when ingesting spicy chilis as capsaicin is an irritant when in contact with skin. Capsaicin has been demonstrated to act against certain types of cancer through apoptosis or programmed cell death. It increases blood flow and acts as an expectorant and bronchodilator. Additionally, capsaicin has been said to activate production of endorphins to reduce pain and produce a sense of well-being.[47]

Radishes

Radishes belong to the cruciferous family, (also called Brassicaceae), named for the cross pattern formed by their leaves. Notable members of this family include cauliflower, cabbage, bok choy and broccoli. Juicing radishes provides a wealth of nutrition in the form of vitamin C, B vitamins, folate, calcium and minerals. The B vitamins present in radishes are known to stabilize the mood. If the B vitamins alone don't lift your mood, knowing that radishes are just as protective against cancers as the members of the cruciferous family may lift your spirits. Studies in rats have demonstrated eradication of cholesterol gallstones, elevation of HDL (good) cholesterol and decrease in triglycerides.[48] These studies in mice seem to support long-standing role in herbal medicine in liver cleansing and gall stone removal. Radishes may be peeled or juiced whole. I prefer to leave the skin on after a thorough washing because much of the nutritional value is concentrated in the skin.

Spinach

Spinach is one of the healthiest foods, rich in protein, iron, vitamins A and K, calcium, folate and is one of the best sources of potassium- a natural substitute for sodium. A single serving of spinach yields over 1000 percent of the daily recommended value of vitamin K, a vital fat soluble molecular associated with bone, blood and protein development.[39] Spinach aids in energy generation through iron and magnesium. Its anti-cancer effects are derived from chlorophyll, vitamins A, K and b-carotene. Cooking spinach is known to unlock more nutritional value than eating it raw; however, juicing provides a means to breakdown the cell wall to unlock the healthy contents. Green smoothies are an excellent vehicle for introducing spinach to your diet and spinach tends to be a popular green for smoothies because of its neutral flavor. The vitamins and minerals such as magnesium and vitamin A are essential for bone and skin health.

Sweet Potato

Sweet potatoes are one of the best sources of B-carotene, are high in vitamin C, the B-vitamins and minerals, such as potassium, magnesium, copper. The great part about juicing sweet potatoes, aside from the sweet creaminess they lend, is that all the nutritional benefits are available to us. Roasting sweet potatoes can destroy the powerful antioxidant combinations like copper/zinc superoxide dismutase and catalase. These super enzyme systems are an important part of our cell's defense mechanism to protect against free radical oxidative damage. When unchecked, oxidative damage can result in cell mutation and ultimately cancer. Additionally, sweet potatoes are full of anthocyanin antioxidants which play a dual role as anti-inflammatory agents. To juice sweet potatoes, wash and peel the outer skin to expose the red meat. Cut into chunks small enough to pass through the chute of the juicer. Cinnamon works well to complement many sweet potato juice recipes.

Tofu (Soy)

Tofu is made by curdling soymilk until it becomes coagulated. It is often called "bean curd". Aside from serving as a vegetarian protein source, mineral rich tofu offers extremely high amounts of calcium, manganese, copper, phosphorus and selenium. Tofu is packed with antioxidants such as flavonoids, phenolic acids, phytosterols. While many forms are tofu are hermetically sealed and do not require refrigeration prior to opening, once opened, tofu should be kept in water and stored refrigerated for up to a week. Change the water daily for maximum freshness.

Tomato

Until the 1600th century, the tomato was mistakenly thought to be poisonous based on its shared membership with the poisonous nightshade family companion, black henbane. Though botanically characterized as a fruit, tomatoes have long since been grouped with vegetables in the United States. Tomatoes are rich in vitamins A, C, K and provide the antioxidant lycopene. Though cooking releases more lycopene than eating raw tomatoes, the benefits of antioxidants like beta-carotene, lutein and lycopene can be enjoyed in raw form as well. After washing, tomatoes can be juiced with the skin intact. They are complimented well by celery, peppers and onion in vegetable juices.

Wheatgrass

Juices made from young, natural grasses are extremely healthy and have become quite popular for juicing. Wheatgrass juice is sold in many places as a shot, and is purported to have a cleansing power, provide an energy boost and confer protective antioxidant effects. Wheatgrass is loaded with chlorophyll, which improves red blood cell function and acts as a powerful antioxidant. There is some evidence suggesting that wheatgrass can aid in binding toxins and clearing them from the body. The Hippocrates Health Institute cites that wheatgrass stimulates the thyroid gland, which can correct obesity and indigestion.[49] By restoring pH levels to neutral through its alkalinity, wheatgrass prevents ulcers, relieves pain and maintains bone health. I was recently following an internet forum entitled, "Wheatgrass-what a disgusting taste." It seems along with the health benefits, the rumors about the "unique" taste of wheatgrass are circling. While wheatgrass will probably not edge out the chocolate milkshake for flavor, there are some ways to improve the taste through combination of wheatgrass juice with other complementary juices. One final advantage is that wheatgrass, like many herbs, can be simply grown in a kitchen herb pot and snipped as needed for addition to juices. Because of the thick cell wall, wheatgrass must be processed in a masticating juicer. A blender or centrifugal juicer will not allow the required breakdown of cell walls to permit efficient extraction of the nutrients.

Herbs, Spices & Roots

Basil

This herb and member of the mint family has played a central role in traditional medicine for centuries for treatment of nausea, headache and anxiety. Depending on the variety, basil may possess a lemony, cinnamon or anise-like flavor. Like many leafy greens, basil leaves contain vitamins A and K, potassium, folate. The phenolic (aromatic) oils are responsible for the antimicrobial, anti-inflammatory and anti-cancer properties. Specifically, camphor and 1,8-cineole are antibacterial; rosmarinic and caffeic acids possess strong antioxidant properties.[36] Researchers at the ETH in Switzerland implicated an organic compound in basil, (E)-beta-caryophyllene in the anti-inflammatory pathway, which may be useful for lessening symptoms of arthritis.Error! Bookmark not defined. Nutritionist and author David Grotto provides some helpful tips for storage and use of basil.[36] While basil may only be stored for several days in the refrigerator, cut stems can be suspended in water in a lighted place, such as a windowsill. Basil leaves may also be layered on wax paper and frozen. Grotto reports that the leaves are likely to darken, but the flavor and aroma remain intact.

Cayenne Pepper

Cayenne pepper is known to break up mucus congestion, redirect pain stimulus to alleviate migraine headaches, detoxify, relieve joint pain, aid in digestion, boost metabolism and stimulate blood circulation. The active ingredient in cayenne pepper is capsaicin, a fiery molecule associated with reduction in musculoskeletal or neuropathic pain. Cayenne pepper additionally promotes tooth and gum health. Add a dash of cayenne pepper to smoothies or juices for extra kick and to reap the benefits indicated above.

Cilantro

Also known as coriander, the cilantro leaf is used as an herb and its seeds are ground and used as a spice. Cilantro offers the rich benefits of vitamins A, C K folate and minerals calcium, iron and magnesium. Its medicinal and healthful benefits span over 8,000 years and are rooted in its digestive, aphrodisiac, anti-fungal and anti-biotic and stimulant properties.[38] The phenolic antioxidants and chlorophyll phytonutrients are responsible for its anticancer effects. Aside from protection against cancer, the high b-carotene content is known to improve vision. It is a natural heavy metal detoxifier when used in juices. Leaves should be bright green and free from yellowing or browning. After washing and removing any discolored or spoiled leaves and stems, the cilantro is best kept wrapped in a damp paper towel, placed in a plastic bag and refrigerated for up to one week.

Cinnamon

Cinnamon has been associated with reduction of blood sugar levels and, as such, has been recommended to Type II diabetics in some cases. Additional healthful benefits of cinnamon include the ability to alleviate stomach and digestive pains, a tendency to freshen breath and maintain gum health, and provide antioxidant protection. Cinnamon tea, prepared by steeping a natural cinnamon stick in boiling water, can be drunk directly or cooled and used as the basis for a smoothie. Cinnamon pairs well with apple, coconut, banana and sweet potatoes in smoothies.

Garlic

The sulfurous compounds responsible for imparting to garlic its characteristic flavor when used in cooking are also thought to deliver a host of therapeutic benefits, so much so that garlic supplements have been catapulted to one of the top selling herbal supplements in the United States. Two particular classes of organosulfur compounds are chiefly found in garlic: (1) gamma-glutamylcysteines, and (2) cysteine sulfoxides.[50] When garlic is crushed, a cascade of complex reactions is set in motion to create from these constituents' new sulfur-containing molecules. It is likely these byproducts which provide cholesterol lowering effects, antioxidant protection, and reduced platelet aggregation (platelet aggregation is associated with blocking of arteries). Studies in China have demonstrated reverse correlations between garlic consumption and gastric and colorectal cancer occurrence (results with other cancers are inconclusive). Garlic may also assist is clearance of toxins through activation of metabolic enzymes charged with destroying xenotoxins (foreign toxins). Garlic has been employed throughout the ages as a natural cold and flu remedy[51] and indeed, several recipes in this book containing garlic are recommend for these ailments. Garlic may be added to vegetable juices and is best blended with powerful or spicy flavors in order not to overpower the juice (see V10, for example). The somewhat overpowering odor can be tempered by eating fresh parsley.

Ginger

Ginger is a member of *Zingiberaceae* family along with its counterpart cardamom, turmeric and galangal, spices predominant in Indian cooking. The rhizome (underground plant stem) may be ground, powdered or extracted into oil for use in cooking or traditional medicine. The National Library of Medicine cites uses of ginger in connection with its treatment of ailments associated with the stomach and digestive system, including motion and morning sickness, diarrhea, nausea and loss of appetite.[52] Ginger is also used to treat arthritis and inflammation and applied locally as a burn treatment. The antibiotic and antifungal properties of ginger combined with its ability to fight inflammation in the gut may be the key to understanding its action to reduce colon cancer. The immune boosting effects of ginger are also well established. Ginger complements apple, lime, beet, spinach, cilantro, fennel and pear. Freezing ginger is an excellent method to keep its freshness for up to six months. Simply apply a rasp to freshly grate the amount needed for your juice or smoothie.

Turmeric

Turmeric[10] is a root, commonly formed into a powder as a base for the flavor and rich yellow color in Indian curry dishes. It has a cleansing effect and can aid in digestion and liver maintenance, serving as an anti-inflammatory and antibacterial agent and as a natural cold and bronchitis herbal medicine. The antioxidant curcuminoids curb damage of oxidative free radicals, inhibit growth of cancer cells and exert a protective effect on the liver.[51] Turmeric is high in minerals present as manganese, potassium and iron and vitamin B6. Because of its strong flavor, turmeric is best

[10] *Quick Tip: Passing turmeric root as one of the first ingredients through the juicer will allow for easier cleaning. The subsequent ingredients will naturally clean the juicer by blending the turmeric oils into the extract.*

combined with beets, carrots or celery and (as in Indian cuisine) matches well with ginger. Curcumin, a phenolic antioxidant, is thought to be the active ingredient in turmeric. Because curcumin is fat-soluble, it is best to combine turmeric with a fatty substance for maximum uptake (think avocado or coconut). Piperine, one of the ingredients in black pepper increases the absorption of turmeric by up to 2000%.

Green Smoothies

Victoria Boutenko, a pioneering raw foods health advocate, is credited with popularizing the green smoothie as an easy and delicious option for consuming large amounts of green, leafy vegetables.[53] As the story goes, Boutenko noted the stark contrast in the diets of chimpanzees, who share over 96% of our DNA,[54] and humans. Our primate cousins consume approximately 40% of their diet in the form of green vegetables, whereas the American diet had a comparative intake of approximately 3% green vegetables. The green smoothie became the experimental vehicle for packing into our diet more greens than we could eat!

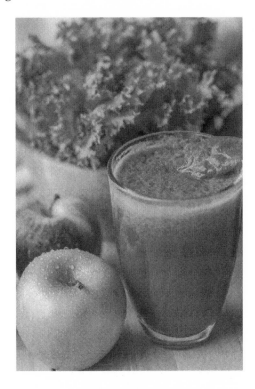

Photo credit: rawpixel

What Makes a Green Smoothie?

In the broadest sense, a green smoothie is a blended drink containing some type of leafy greens, some liquid and, for the right consistency, a creamy complement like banana, mango, pineapple, avocado or kiwi. There are endless varieties and the resulting smoothie need not even be green!   With respect to greens, I recommend beginning with spinach, because it keeps well, can be found pre-washed in nearly every grocery store and has a mild flavor easily compatible with fruits and vegetables. Spinach is also easily blended and doesn't require processing through a juicer like wheatgrass. Realistically, any green can play the central role of leafy green in a green smoothie. Some typical greens organized by their strength (i.e. pungency or bitterness) are indicated below.

Mild Greens	Strong Greens
Spinach	Mustard greens
Kale	Parsley
Dandelion greens	Cilantro
Beet greens	Wheatgrass
Romaine lettuce	Fennel greens
Swiss chard	

Several excellent resources are available offering recipes for green smoothies, including Kristine Mills' The Green Smoothie Bible[55] and Victoria Boutenko's Green for Life: The Updated Classic on Green Smoothie Nutrition.[56]

Let's dissect the components of my typical green smoothie (**Original Green Smoothie**) to better understand the powerful benefits of introducing the green smoothie into your breakfast or midday snack:

©2018 Kevin Finn

The ingredients: orange juice, spinach, pineapple, parsley, apple, celery, chia seeds, ginger[11]

Orange Juice (8 Oz)

- Provides 100% of daily recommended supply of vitamin C; soluble fiber, B vitamins, potassium and flavonoids

Spinach (1 cup loosely packed)

- High in iron, calcium and rich in antioxidants such as chlorophyll and lutein. Flavonoid rich. Serves to raise the pH of the blood to prevent leaching of calcium from bones

Pineapple (1/2 cup)

- Contains bromelain, a natural enzyme aiding in digestion and associated with reducing inflammation. Provides vitamin C, B vitamins, and minerals such as copper, manganese, magnesium and fiber.

Parsley (1 Tbsp)

- Rich source of chlorophyll, a compound associated with improving blood function and detoxification; provides vitamin C, folate and trace minerals

Apple (1 green apple, cored)

---

[11] *Quick Tip: Ginger can be stored up to six months in the freezer. Frozen ginger is also easier to grate!*

- Apples are high in vitamin C, antioxidant flavonoids, potassium, fiber and pectin.

<u>Chia Seeds (1 tsp)</u>

- Chia seeds yield high amounts of plant-derived protein and antioxidants.

<u>Ginger (1 tsp, grated frozen)</u>

- The anti-inflammatory, nausea-reducing and immune boosting properties of ginger are well established.

The total complement of the green breakfast smoothie surpasses the recommended daily value of vitamin C (orange, pineapple, parsley, apple), provides antioxidant and anticancer protection (oranges, spinach, parsley, apples, chia seeds), reduces cholesterol through pectin (apples), provides joint and pain relief via anti-inflammatory compounds (pineapple, ginger), reduces blood pressure by increasing blood potassium levels (orange, apple) and improves bone structure through increased blood pH and calcium supply (spinach). Not to mention, the fiber gives the drink substances to last until the next meal. By rotating the greens, sweet fruits, supplements and base juices, the health benefit combinations are nearly endless.

The pH Effect

In his best-selling book "Beating Cancer with Nutrition",[57] Dr. Patrick Quillin stresses the importance of maintaining proper acid-base balance in the body. The pH scale, spanning from 1-14 refers to the spectrum of acidity (low pH) or basicity (high pH) in water or blood. Neutral pH is 7. Vegetables and other plant foods promote a healthy alkaline or basic pH profile, which tends toward slightly higher range in the bloodstream. Foods associated with an unhealthy pH effect (more acidic) include meat, dairy and sugar. Dr. Quillin goes on to explain that cancer cells release lactic acid during their growth. This pH-lowering process, termed the Cori cycle, hampers the cell's ability to combat cancer. Infections and cancer both compromise the body's natural immune response. It may seem quite counterintuitive, but foods which are naturally acidic prior to ingestion become alkaline in the body. Examples of these foods include tomatoes and lemons. Alkaline-producing foods found in these recipes are spinach, kale, oranges, apples.

Figure 7: Blood pH Spectrum and Health

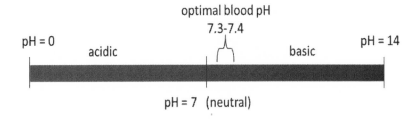

Lemon and Water

One of the simplest and most effective ways to detoxify the body, increase immune response and promote weight loss is consumption of warm water with lemon. It may surprise you to learn that, although lemon juice is acidic in water, it is alkaline in the body. Because the human body is always slightly alkaline (excepting certain organs like the stomach), an overall alkaline pH is better for your body. Joe Cross, whom we have met in the section on Juice

Fasts, suggests drinking warm water with lemon in the morning and in the evening during the fast.

Original Green Smoothie

This old standby was the first smoothie recipe I developed and still faithfully use nearly every day. The filling nature of oatmeal or protein powder may be added to make the morning smoothie stretch until lunch. I find this smoothie provides me a fresh, energizing start to each day. You may want to employ the following time saving tricks to ensure the morning smoothie fits into your routine: (1) pre-cutting and freezing the pineapple; (2) purchasing pre-washed "juicing greens", normally consisting of swiss chard, spinach and kale (alternatively you may make your own mixture and wash in advance); (3) pre-mixing protein powder, chia seeds and oatmeal in the desired proportion.

12 fl oz orange juice

½ cup pineapple (see Quick Tip)

0.5 oz washed and de-stemmed kale (about 1 stalk)

1 cup spinach

1 granny smith apple (core removed)

1 stalk celery

1 tsp grated ginger

1 tsp chia seeds

1 tbsp vanilla vegan pea protein powder (optional)

1 Tbsp oatmeal or flaxseed (optional)

Makes 4 cups

Cactus Smoothie

8 oz orange juice

1 cup sliced and prepared* prickly pear cactus (2 medium sized paddles)

2 cups pineapple chunks

2.5 oz cucumber

3 oz strawberries

0.5 cup ice[12]

Makes 4 cups

---

[12] *Quick Tip: Instead of adding ice, freeze fruits beforehand. Works great for pineapple chunks and berries.*

Cleveland Clinic Green Grape Smoothie Recipe[58]

The following recipe is found on the website of the world-famous Cleveland Clinic, a center of excellence for cancer research, treatment and prevention. The Cleveland Clinic touts this as a delicious smoothie with "cancer-fighting greens to keep you going."

1 cup cleaned spinach leaves, firmly packed

1 cup cleaned kale, roughly chopped, firmly packed

1 cup green seedless grapes

1 Bartlett pear – core, stem and seeds removed

1 orange – peeled, pith removed, quartered

1 banana– peeled

1 teaspoon chia seeds

½ cup water

2 cups ice

Place all ingredients in blender. Process on low speed for 15 seconds. Increase to medium speed, then high speed. Process until well blended.

Makes 5, 8 oz servings

Luminous Skin Smoothie

1 cup orange juice

5 oz pineapple

1 tsp cilantro

1 lime, squeezed

1 ripe avocado

1 Granny Smith apple

1 cup ice

Makes 4 cups

Banana Blueberry

8 oz orange juice

3 oz pineapple

½ banana

2 oz blueberries

1 oz spinach

Blend thoroughly; yields 2 cups

Creamy Green Banana Smoothie

8 oz orange juice

2 oz pineapple

½ banana

½ avocado

Tsp chia seeds

1 in cucumber

1 Kale leaf

1 oz spinach

Blend until smooth; makes 2 cups

Beet Green Smoothie

1 small beet, peeled

1 cup orange juice

1 orange, peeled

2 cups spinach or beet greens

½ lemon juices

6 oz strawberries

1 tsp ginger

Guava Green

1 cup orange juice

½ cup chilled water

4 oz pineapple

1 Tbsp cilantro

½ nopal paddle (prepared as described in Cactus Subsection)

1 oz spinach

3 strawberry guavas

1 kiwi

3 oz cucumber

Juice of 1 lime

Makes 3 cups

Green Pear Smoothie

11 oz coconut water

1 lime, juiced

1 green pear

1 oz spinach

3 oz cucumber, peeled

©2018 Kevin Finn

1 green apple

1 tsp basil leaves

Makes 3.5 cups

Melon Kale

8 oz orange juice

1 cup watermelon

4 kale leaves

1 pear

Makes 3 cups

Coconut Clementine Green Smoothie[59]

This delicious smoothie is courtesy of chef blogger, recipe creator and food photographer Minimalist Baker. [60]

4-5 clementine

1 ripe banana (sliced and frozen)

½ light coconut milk

1 cup greens

3 or 4 ice cubes

2-3 mint leaves

Blend all ingredients until smooth; for added sweetness, put additional banana, makes 3 ½ cups

Dandelion Green Smoothie[61]

Dandelions are as bitter as they are healthy, and we have adapted this recipe to allow for a little more sweetness to offset the powerful taste of dandelions.

1 cup water

1 cup chopped dandelion greens

1 banana

1 cup fresh or frozen blueberries

1 tbsp vanilla vegan pea protein powder

For added sweetness, use ½ cup water and ½ cup fresh orange juice. Blend all ingredients until smooth and creamy.

Kiwi Melon Green Smoothie

2 cups swiss chard

2 cups watermelon

3 oz cucumber

1 cup water

2 oz freshly squeezed lemon juice

1 kiwi

Blend thoroughly; makes 3 ½ cups

Shauna's Carrot Cake Smoothie[62]

2 cups fresh spinach

1 ½ cups coconut mile

1 cup pineapple

2 pears

1 banana

½ inch piece ginger

Makes 3 cups

Fruit Smoothies

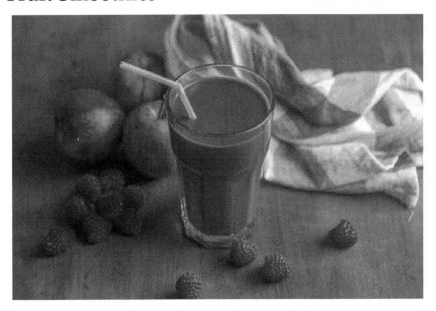

Mango Berry

A great tasting smoothie with antioxidant power to repair damaged skin with the pore cleansing capabilities of mango.

1 cup water

2 oz raspberries

2 oz blackberries

2 oz blueberries

1 ripe mango (seed removed)

1 tsp chia seeds

Makes 2.5 cups

Watermelon Cooler

Watermelon makes an excellent base for a smoothie and will keep you well-hydrated on those scorching August days. Do you have leftover watermelon from Sunday's barbecue taking up an entire shelf of your refrigerator? Let's put it to good use in this easy recipe featuring watermelon, lime and strawberries. Aside from its hydrating properties, the ingredients in this smoothie confer protective benefits against cancer, inflammation and indigestion. A summary of their individual healthy attributes is described below.

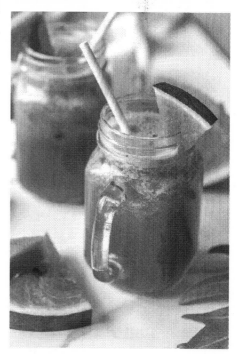

2 cups watermelon

1 lime, juiced

1/2 cup strawberries, sliced

1/2 cup ice

Blend all ingredients until smooth. Garnish with basil or mint.

Blue Melon

2 cups watermelon

1 cup blueberries

½ cup crushed ice

Yields 3 ½ cups

Super Berry

1 1/3 cups freshly-squeezed orange juice

2 oz raspberries

2 oz blackberries

2 oz blueberries

0.5 cup water

For extra energy, add 1 oz spinach

Makes 4 cups

Orange-Cantaloupe

4 fl oz carrot juice

3 oz cantaloupe

4 oz pineapple

3 oz strawberries

1 tsp chia seeds

Makes 2.5 cups

Mango-Coconut

8 fl oz orange juice

1 mango, sliced

1 oz fresh coconut slices

1 cup ice

4 fl oz chilled water

1 pinch cinnamon

Makes 3 cups

Peach Berry

2.5 oz blueberries

1 kiwi

2 peaches, deseeded

Juice of 1 lemon (approximately 2 oz)

3 oz strawberries

0.5 cup orange juice

1.5 cup ice

Makes 4 cups

Beet & Berry

1 cup chopped raw, peeled beets

½ cup strawberries

½ cup blueberries

1 banana

1 cup soy or coconut milk

1 tsp grated ginger

Pinch cinnamon

1 tsp chia seeds (optional) for additional protein

Mango Papaya Morning Start

1 cup orange juice

2 oz carrot juice

10 oz papaya, peeled and deseeded

4 oz mango, sliced

4 oz pineapple

0.5 oz coconut meat

2 tsp chia seeds

1 cup crushed ice

Makes 4 cups

Pineapple-Kiwi-Coconut

10 oz pineapple

1 Granny Smith Apple (peeled)

1 kiwi

11 oz coconut water

Blend and serve

Makes 4 cups

Berry Coconut Water Smoothie

11 oz coconut water

3/4 cup blackberries

2 cups strawberries

2 kiwis

Makes 3.5 cups

Pomegranate Mango

The juice of pomegranates is well worth the trouble to harvest. Some of my favorite juices in this book are derived from pomegranate, which is linked with good heart health. This juice provides an antioxidant boost in the form of orange juice, pomegranate and chia seeds.

6 oz pomegranate juice (or juice of two pomegranates)

6 oz orange juice (or juice of one orange)

1 mango

1 kiwi

tsp chia seeds

0.5 cup skim milk

Makes 3 cups

Jam Master Juice (aka Joseph Persimmons)

1 persimmon

1.5 cup ice

1 lime, juiced

1 orange, juiced

5 oz strawberries

1 green apple

Makes 3 cups

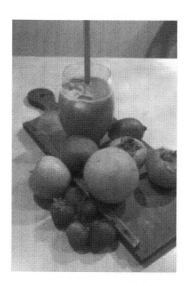

Passion Fruit Watermelon

Contents of 2 passion fruits

8 oz watermelon juice

1 nectarine

Blend with 0.5 cup crushed ice

Makes 2 cups

Guava Fruit

8 oz orange juice

4 oz skim milk

1 kiwi

3 oz strawberry

3.5 oz pineapple

1 guava

Makes 3 cups

Guava Mango

1 cup orange juice

½ cup skim milk

1 yellow mango

3 strawberry guavas

Makes 2 cups

Mango Beet

1 lb. beet root

1 orange, juiced

1 large carrot

Process beet, orange and carrot in juicer; yields 16 oz; transfer into blender with:

1 mango, sliced and core removed

1 cup ice

1 tsp ginger

Blend thoroughly

Makes 4 cups

Lychee-Pineapple Cooler

7-8 lychees, peeled and pitted

5 oz pineapple

1 cup chilled water

1 cup crushed ice

Pinch cinnamon

Blend well; makes 2.5 cups

Berry Fiber

8 oz orange juice

5 oz pineapple

4 oz strawberries

3 oz blueberries

½ cactus paddle

1 oz spinach

1 green apple

1 Tbsp oats

1 tsp chia seeds

½ cup chilled water

Mango Plum

1 cup chilled water

3 large plums, pit removed

1 mango

6 lychees

1.5 oz spinach

Makes 4 cups

Cactus Pear Strawberry Cooler

Cactus pear provides a host of beneficial antioxidants and tart flavor that combines wonderfully with fresh orange. The lychee provides added sweetness and spinach allows you to feel even better about enjoying this sweet treat.

8 oz orange juice

4 cactus pears

6 oz strawberries

5 lychees

1.5 cup spinach

½ cup crushed ice

Blend thoroughly, makes 3.5 cups

Blueberry-Pear Smoothie

½ cup chilled water

8 oz blueberries

3 oz pineapple (or more for sweeter taste)

1 oz spinach

1 pear

3 oz plain yogurt

½ cup crushed ice

Makes 3 cups

Clementine-Strawberry

4 clementine, peeled and juiced (8 oz)

1 apple, juiced (4 oz)

6-7 oz strawberries

2 oz blueberries

4 oz tofu

Add strawberries, blueberries and tofu to juice mixture;

blend thoroughly; makes 3 cups

Tropical Beet

6 oz beet juice

6 oz orange juice

6 oz water

4 oz pineapple

1 mango, peeled and cored

Pinch of cilantro

1 cup dandelion greens

Blend until smooth; makes 3 cups

Guava Strawberry Green Tea

4 guavas

2 cups chilled green tea

1 cup strawberries

1 tsp sugar

Process guava with green tea in blender. Filter through a screen to remove guava seeds. Introduce filtered liquid in the blender with 1/2 cup of strawberries and 1/2 tsp honey. Blend until smooth. Makes 2.5 cups.

Banana Strawberry Kiwi

The ingredients for this creamy, delicious smoothie are available year-round and blend easily.

8 oz orange juice

½ banana

2 kiwis

3 oz strawberries

½ cup ice

Blend thoroughly; makes 2 ½ cups

Mango Banana Kiwi

16 oz orange juice

1 mango

1 banana

2 kiwis

2 oz blueberries

1 cup crushed ice

Makes 3.5 cups

Fall Strawberry Persimmon

8 oz soy milk

1 Fuyu persimmon

7 oz strawberries

Dash cinnamon

Handful of ice

Blend thoroughly; makes 2.5 cups

Aloevita Tropical Smoothie

I created this delicious tropical concoction to share with my Dad when he was undergoing radiation and chemotherapy. My Dad's oncologist prescribed a daily tablespoon dose of aloe preparation to aid in his healing following radiation treatment. Aloe is one natural medication which quickly degrades unless stabilized with preservatives. I decided to create a fresh aloe combination to avoid

preservatives and counter the typical bitter taste of aloe. The coconut water base is intended to hydrate and introduce electrolytes, the aloe aids in skin repair, the coconut meat provides fiber and calories. The mango and pineapple yield vitamin C and provide a sweet and fruity tropical flavor.

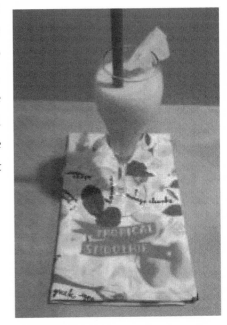

8 oz frozen pineapple chunks

1 large ripe mango, peeled and deseeded

1 cup of fresh Thai coconut water

2 oz fresh Thai coconut flesh

½ cup aloe vera pulp, obtained by "fileting" 1 whole aloe vera leaf

Blend thoroughly; yields 3.5 cups

Fall Strawberry Persimmon Smoothie

8 oz soy milk

2 Fuyu persimmons

7 oz strawberries

Dash cinnamon

Handful of ice

Blend thoroughly; makes 2.5 cups

Fresh Juices

In addition to the recipes found below, several books have been dedicated to juicing.[63]

including.

Cilantro-Celery-Ginger

6 oz fresh celery juice

2 oz fresh cilantro (processed in juicer)

Squeezed lemon

1 tsp grated ginger

Orange-Pineapple-Celery-Carrot

2 oz carrot juice

2 oz orange juice

2 oz celery juice

2 oz pineapple juice

Orange Dreamsicle[64]

This creamy orange juice is based on a similar concoction from JuiceRecipes.com. One of my favorite morning juices (and one of the best after a long night), the Orange Dreamsicle is a mélange of sweet orange, creamy sweet potato, mildly sweet apple and pear with a hint of celery and ginger. Although not included in the original recipe, I prefer to add a bit of ginger for taste and added immune system benefit.

1 green apple

1 stalk celery

1 orange, peeled

1 pear

1 sweet potato

½ tsp fresh ginger

Makes 24 oz juice

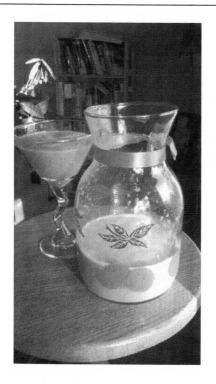

Beet-Carrot-Pineapple

10 oz beet, peeled

10 oz carrots, peeled (should add less)

3 oz pineapple (should add more)

¼ tsp turmeric

pinch black pepper

¼ tsp ginger

Makes 1.5 cups

Mango Coconut Pineapple

1 mango

1 oz coconut

3 oz pineapple

5 oz fresh coconut milk

Pinch cinnamon

Makes 12 oz

Pomegranate-Lime

Juice from 2 pomegranates, deseeded (approximately 2 cups seeds)

2 oz grapefruit juice

2 oz lime juice

3 oz orange juice

Makes 12 oz juice

Vitamin C Supercharge

½ grapefruit

1 apple

Pinch parsley

1 kiwi

5 oz pineapple

1 orange

Juice all ingredients

Makes 20 oz juice

Cucumber-Apple

½ cucumber

6 oz pineapple

1 Granny Smith apple

1 stalk celery

1/4 cup ice

Makes 2 cups

Pomegranate Kiwi

Seeds from 2 pomegranates (approximately 2 cups

3 kiwis

Juice all ingredients and serve over ice

Makes 8 oz

Beet Carrot Apple

3 oz beet juice

3 oz carrot juice

3 oz apple juice

Tsp shaved ginger

Persimmon-Kiwi-Apple

Here is a great Autumn recipe.

2 medium sized persimmons

1 large Granny Smith apple

1 kiwi

Juice all ingredients

Dilute with ½ cup chilled water

Makes 2 cups

Purple Viking

2 oz spinach

3 oz blackberries

3 oz blueberries

3 oz raspberries

1 Granny Smith apple

Juice all ingredients; add ½ cup grapefruit juice and ¾ cup beet juice

Introduce to blender and mix well. Serve over ice

Makes 3 cups

Orange Sunrise

One of the best ways to begin the day, the Orange Sunrise provides a great introduction to fresh juices for those just getting started.

1 orange, peeled

5 oz carrot, peeled

8 oz pineapple

Juice all ingredients separately, mix in shaker

Makes 1.5 cups

Peach Orange Delight

5-6 carrots

1 peach, pitted

½ cup pineapple

1-inch ginger

Juice all ingredients and pour over ice

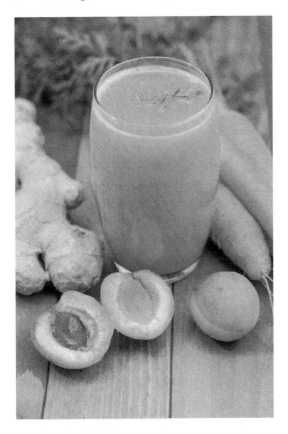

©2018 Kevin Finn

Apple Berry Lemonade

3.5 oz raspberries

3.5 oz blueberries

3.5 oz blackberries

2 Granny Smith apples

1 lemon

Juice all ingredients; mix and serve

Makes 18 oz

The Eye Doctor

15 oz peeled and deseeded papaya (yields approximately 8 oz juice)

2 Granny Smith apples (yields approximately 6 oz juice)

6 oz pineapple (yields 3 oz juice)

4 oz carrot juice

Pinch lemon zest

Juice all ingredients, add 1 cup ice

Blend and serve

Makes 3 cups

Beet Carrot Apple Celery

1 small beet

10 oz carrot

2 stalks celery

1 oz spinach

1 Granny Smith apple

Pinch turmeric

Pinch cayenne pepper

Makes 12 oz

Starfruit Sorpresa

1 starfruit

5 oz cucumber (less next time)

1 mango

Juice all ingredients; add 6 oz coconut water

Makes 16 oz

Cactus Pear Cooler

4 cactus pears, peeled

1.5 oz cucumber

Lime

Juice all ingredients; add ½ cup coconut water and serve over ice

Makes 10 oz

Cactus Kiwi Orange

1 kiwi

2 oranges, peeled[13]

4 cactus pears, prepared as described in Section X

Juice all ingredients

Chill and serve

Makes 2 cups

Cactus Sunrise

1 kiwi

---

[13] *Quick Tip: Juice oranges can be more difficult to peel than Navel or Valencia. A handy trick for peeling oranges is to remove the top and bottom sections with a sharp knife. A single cut down the middle will allow you to unfold the orange and expose the inner segments for easy processing.*

1 orange, peeled[14]

3cactus pears, prepared as described below

1 pear, pealed

Juice all ingredients

Chill and serve

Makes 12 oz

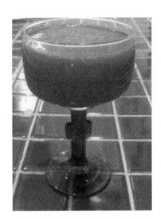

---

[14] *Quick Tip: Juice oranges can be more difficult to peel than Navel or Valencia. A handy trick for peeling oranges is to remove the top and bottom sections with a sharp knife. A single cut down the middle will allow you to unfold the orange and expose the inner segments for easy processing.*

Grapefruit Nectarine

1 grapefruit (8-10 oz juice)

3 nectarines

Juice all ingredients

Makes 14 oz

Pomegranate Grape Juice

2 pomegranates (1 cup seeds, 4 oz juice)

3 oranges, juiced (12 oz)

5 oz seedless black grapes

Makes 16 oz

Grape Strawberry Juice

10 oz grapes, (8 oz juice)

5 oz strawberries

1 green apple

16 oz

Beet-Grapefruit-Orange

1 1 lb. beet, peeled and juiced

1 grapefruit, peeled and juiced

1 orange, peeled and juiced

Sweet Beet

1 lb. beet root

1 orange, juiced

1 large carrot

Process beet, orange and carrot in juicer; yields 16 oz;

Clementine-Apple

4 medium clementine, peeled

1 Granny Smith apple

Juice ingredients separately and mix thoroughly afterward

Makes 12 oz

Beet Mixture

3 six oz beets

0.5 oz parsley

2 stalks red kale

2 kiwis

1 Granny Smith apple

2 tsp ginger

Makes 20 oz

Spicy Hot V10 Vegetable Juice

I love Spicy Hot® V-8 blend, but the high sodium and pasteurization processing detract from its natural goodness. This recipe is my own take on Spicy Hot® V-8. I've added a couple of extra ingredients to round out the taste and maximize the health benefits. Additionally, the spice level can be tuned through substitution depending on your preference or sensitivity. The high vitamin C, decongestive power of chili and onion combined with the traditional cold remedying effects of garlic render this an indispensable natural cold treatment. For extra kick to combat congestion, substitute a chili powder for a fresh jalapeño or habeñero pepper. Do so at your own comfort and risk level!

(least spicy)
Cayenne powder <
jalapeño pepper <
habeñero pepper
    (spiciest)

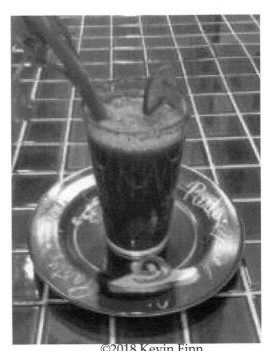

3 large carrots

2 cups spinach

0.5 oz parsley

1 small beet

3 stalks celery

4 oz cucumber

©2018 Kevin Finn

1 clove garlic

1 small green bell pepper

1 spring onion

1 small lemon, peeled

Pinch cayenne

2 Roma tomatoes

Dash powdered cayenne pepper or 1 habeñero pepper (optional-for extra spice). Introduce all ingredients sequentially into the juicer. If using cayenne powder, add this separately to the prepared juice. If using fresh chili pepper, juice along with other vegetables.

Captain Chlorophyll

Absolutely dominating in chlorophyllation, this juice is great for the blood and skin.

2 cups baby spinach

1 cups freshly clipped wheatgrass

6 stalks celery

1 medium sized cucumber, peeled

Juice of 1 lime

Juice spinach, wheatgrass, celery and cucumber sequentially. Add lime juice. Filter through a strainer to remove foam. Makes 20 oz

Tart Berry Currant

If you love sour, you're going to love this concoction. Currants are loaded with antioxidant phytochemicals and vitamin C. A little sweetness is needed to balance the tartness, but feel free to substitute honey or Stevia for the raw sugar.

6 oz red currants

6 oz raspberries

6 oz strawberries

1 green apple

Pinch sugar

Juice all ingredients; add to 16 oz sparkling water; makes 32 oz

Top Tummy

2 large carrots, peeled

1 fennel bulb

2 celery stalks

2 tsp grated ginger

Juice the carrots, fennel and celery stalks. Add ginger to the juice mixture. Makes 14 oz.

Wheatgrass-Mango-Cactus Pear

0.5 oz freshly cut wheatgrass

2 mangos, peeled

4 cactus pears, peeled

3 oz pineapple

Juice all ingredients; add to blender containing 2 cups crushed ice. Blend to give 3.5 cups

Green Liver Tonic

6 stalks dandelion greens

1 cup spinach

Pinch of parsley

4 stalks of celery

1 large cucumber (skin on if unwaxed)

1 Granny Smith apple

1 lime, peeled

Juice all ingredients, filter to remove excess foam; add 1 tsp freshly grated ginger;

Makes 24 oz

Morning Green Energy

4 red kale leaves

2 medium carrots

4 celery stalks

1 medium beet

1 green apple

Juice all ingredients sequentially; makes 14 oz

Simple Cherry Juice

Sometimes, simple is best. A you cannot go wrong with fresh cherries. They are loaded with antioxidants and anti-inflammatory compounds and known to be especially good for joint health. Cherries can be overpoweringly sweet, so dilution is recommended.

1 lb. black cherries

Remove the pits by slicing in half and separating the fruit from the pit; process all fruit in the juicer; yields 12 oz juice. Dilute with 12 oz filtered or sparkling water and enjoy.

Total Health Cleanser

3 stalks red kale

2 oz cilantro

2 carrots

4 oz cherry tomatoes

2 garlic cloves

1 jalapeño pepper (seeds and inner membrane removed) Caution- HOT![15]

2 celery stalks

1 lime, whole (sliced to fit into juicer)

Juice all ingredients, dilute with 4 oz chilled water and filter to remove pulp and foam. Makes 20 oz

Detoxifying Radish Blend

I will admit that this recipe is a far cry from tasting like cotton candy, but I trust the healthy glow and good conscience you'll gain after drinking this health tonic will offset the off-putting taste. Radishes are potent liver detoxifiers and act to reduce blood pressure. Cilantro, in turn, is a blood detoxifier. Aside from tempering the pungent taste of the radish, apples provide vitamin C and A and soluble fiber. Finally, cucumbers refresh and rejuvenate the skin and connective tissues.

2 apples

1 cup radishes, skin on

½ cucumber, peeled

Handful of cilantro

Juice all ingredients, add juice of ½ lime; Makes 16 oz

---

[15] *Quick Tip: Remove seeds from jalapeño peppers to temper the spice level*

Vegetable Cleanser

1 large beet, peeled (about 15 oz)

2 medium carrots, peeled

1 stalk celery

5 oz radishes, peeled

1 jalepeño pepper, deveined and seeds removed

1 Roma tomato

Process all ingredients in juicer; filter to remove excess pulp and foam; makes 24 oz

Green Orange Fennel Juice

1 cup spinach

4 large kale leaves

1 cucumber, peeled unless organic and unwaxed

¾ fennel bulb

2 oranges

Process ingredients sequentially in juicer; transfer to blender with 0.5 cup ice and mix thoroughly. Makes 3 cups

Spicy Fennel Beet

¼ fennel bulb

2 ½ oz radishes

3 carrots

1 beet

Juice all ingredients; makes 13 oz

Pineapple Carrot Super Root

4 carrots

1 sweet potato, peeled

1-inch ginger, peeled

4 oz pineapple

Process all ingredients through juicer; makes 12 oz; dilute with 12 oz chilled water to reduce sweetness

Super Beet Cleanser

1 medium beet

1 medium cucumber

4 swiss chard leaves

1 clove garlic

2 small or 1 large apple

Makes 12 oz.

Fennel-Beet

½ *fennel bulb*

1 *apple*

1 *pear*

4 *swiss chard leaves*

1 *beet*

Juice all ingredients; makes 15 oz juice

Cucumber Lemon Cooler

A refreshing summertime favorite with some real pep.

1 *cucumber, peeled if waxed; unpeeled if organic and unwaxed*

1 *lemon peeled*

3 *Tbsp cilantro (optional)*

Juice all ingredients; makes 12 oz juice. Dilute with 6 oz chilled water and enjoy

Cucumber Beet

Greens from one fennel

1 medium beet, peeled

3 carrots

2 celery stalks

1 cucumber, whole

Makes 22 oz

Orange Vegetable Juice

1 sweet potato

3 Tbsp cilantro

1 zucchini, peeled

1 cucumber, whole

4 celery stalks

1 clove garlic

Juice all ingredients; add pinch of cayenne powder to taste; Makes 22 oz

Pineapple Cucumber-Guava

3 strawberry guavas

©2018 Kevin Finn

¼ *pineapple*

1 *cucumber, peeled*

Feed all ingredients through juicer; makes 22 oz

Beet Grapefruit

1 *beet*

1 *pear*

1 *grapefruit*

0.5 *oz wheatgrass*

Juice all ingredients; add ½ tsp fresh ginger; makes 20 oz

Sweet Orange Sunrise

0.5 *oz wheatgrass*

3 *oranges, peeled*

1 *small cucumber*

1 *beet*

1 *pear*

Juice all ingredients; makes 25 oz

Fennel Radish Cleanser

½ *Fennel bulb and stalks*

1 *celery stalk*

5-6 large carrots

6 red radishes, tops removed

Juice all ingredients; add juice of ½ lime; makes 22 oz.

Heart Healer

1 cucumber

1 pear

Handful of mint leaves

1 fennel bulb and stalks

1 celery stalk

Makes 12 oz

Inflammation Fighter

2 inches peeled turmeric root

Pinch parsley

1 stalk kale

1 cup spinach

1 beet

3 carrots

1 orange

1 apple –or– ½ cup purple or black grapes

Makes 20 oz

Purple Inflammation Fighter

1 cup blueberries

1 cup black grapes

1 cup spinach

1 stalk kale (approximately 1 loosely-packed cup)

1 green apple, peeled

Makes 16 oz juice

Salsa in a Glass[65]

1 lime, peeled

1 tomato

½ cucumber, peeled

½ cup cilantro

1 small slice onion

Juice all ingredients; add dash of hot sauce to taste. Makes 8 oz

Mexican Gazpacho

Not to be confused with the cold Spanish tomato soup having the same name, Mexican gazpacho is a fruit salad featuring mango, pineapple, jicama, lime juice with a hefty dose of Tajin® spice. When the fruit is eaten, the tail end of the gazpacho mixture is a slightly salty and spicy lime-flavored fruit juice. This juice is a recreation of the classic refreshing Mexican staple.

2 Manilla mangos, peeled 14 oz

Pineapple, 13 oz

2 small Jicama, peeled (12 oz)

3 limes, juiced

Process mango, pineapple and jicama in juicer. Add lime juice. Season with 1 tsp Tajin®, or similar Mexican spice to taste. Makes 30 oz.

Cucumber, Carrot and Beet[66]

3 carrots

½ cucumber

½ beet with greens

Garden Variety[66]

6-8 tomatoes

3-4 green onions

2 carrots

2 stalks celery

½ green pepper

½ bunch spinach

½ bunch parsley

Cold Combat

1 white grapefruit

1 cup pineapple

2 Bartlett pears

1 tsp ginger, grated.

Juice all fruits; add grated ginger to mixture. Yields 16 oz juice.

Island Punch

This versatile natural punch recipe is a hit as healthy party punch recipe and makes a wonderful homemade Popsicles for the kids.

1 cup cherries, pitted and stems removed

5 oz pineapple

1 green apple

1 mango

Juice all ingredients; makes 16 oz. Add ice and sparkling water

Super Green Zinger

2 cups loosely packed spinach

1 cup loosely packed kale

1 inch of ginger, peeled

4 celery stalks

1 orange, peeled

1 lemon (washed, but unpeeled)

4 green apples, peeled

1 green pear

Juice all ingredients; makes 30 oz

Natural Baby Foods

An increasing number of masticating juicers can prepare baby foods. You will be satisfied to know that you are preparing your child's first foods from natural ingredients you select, free from preservatives, gums, starches, thickening agents and other unwanted ingredients. The entire spectrum of fruits and vegetables and textures can be explored, providing your child with natural, easily digestible foods prepared in your kitchen. There are some cautionary notes to consider, however. Because infant's digestive systems are more sensitive than older children's or adult's, it is imperative to avoid the introduction of bacteria. Here are some guidelines to follow:

1) Work in an extremely clean environment, meticulously cleaning all working surfaces, utensils and the juicer before beginning

2) Use organic produce to minimize exposure to pesticides

3) Carefully wash the outside of the fruits and vegetables; a quick wash in a dilute solution of baking soda is an effective way to clean. It is important to clean the outside even though skins will be removed to prevent accidental contamination of the inner fruit with chemicals from the skin

4) Remove skins and seeds from fruits and vegetables as these are more difficult to digest

5) As an extra precaution, some recommend cooking the vegetables to ensure that bacteria are destroyed. While all cooking methods will kill bacteria, steaming the fruits or vegetables will preserve the most nutrients.

6) Chop the foods into pieces which can be introduced into the chute of the juicer

7) Dilute the foods with water or breast milk to reduce the sweetness and to provide a familiar taste

8) Use the foods immediately to avoid bacterial contamination.

Supplements like wheat germ or flax seed can be conveniently added to vegetable purees. Generally, juices are not recommended before the child's six month. Juices should be slowly added to the child's diet. Juices should be adequate diluted to avoid consumption of excess sugar and should never be given in a bottle, but rather a cup at meal times.

Purees

Apricots

Introduce one Apricot, deseeded, into the juicer. Serve within 24 h for maximum freshness. Makes 3 oz.

Juices

Carrot Juice

Process chopped carrots in a juicer. Dilute juice with 10 parts water prior to serving.

Apple Juice

Place ½ apple through the juicer and dilute resulting juice with 10 parts water.

Smoothies

There are several great resources on the web for preparing your child's smoothies. I've found www.homemade-baby-food-recipes.com[67] to be an excellent resource whose recipes come directly from its readers all over the world. As always, these should be used as a guide, paying special attention to your child's stage of development and considering any food sensitivities your child may have. Most recommend introducing one new fruit at a time to better acclimate your child to new tastes and textures. Smoothies should be prepared and served immediately after processing.

Nutritionist, blogger, author and mother Megan Gilmore shared published many excellent recipes for children's first smoothies. Mrs. Gilmore recipes incorporate at least three elements in each recipe: fruits, greens and fats. These delicious smoothies are found on https://detoxinista.com/ but a sampling of these and flavor for how these components can be combined is presented below. The full details of preparation are available at no charge from Ms. Gilmore's site.

Apple Cinnamon[68]

1 cup water

1 Fuji apple

¼ avocado

2 Medjool dates, pitted

Sprinkle of ground cinnamon

4 large Romaine leaves

Orange Basil

1 cup water

1 navel orange, peeled

2 Medjool dates, pitted

Small handful fresh basil

¼ avocado

½ tsp alcohol-free vanilla

Cherry Berry

1 cup water

½ cup frozen sweet cherries

½ frozen strawberries

2 cups fresh spinach

¼ cup young Thai coconut meat

½ tsp alcohol-free vanilla

Banana Smoothie

1 banana, chopped

¼ cup curd or yogurt

¼ cup water or orange juice (depending on desired sweetness)

Mango Lassi Smoothie

1 whole mango

1/2 cup (4 oz) of plain organic yogurt

Pinch of nutmeg (or cinnamon)

1/4 cup (2 fl oz) of organic milk

Strawberry Smoothie

2 cups strawberries(chopped very small)

1/4 cup (2 fl. oz) prepared milk (I use formula for this)

1 cup (8 fl oz) yogurt

infant apple juice

ice

Banana-Berry Treat

1 ripe banana

1 1/2 cups (approx. 12 oz) favorite frozen berries (blueberries, strawberries, raspberries, blackberries)

1 cup (8 oz) plain yogurt

1/2 cup (4 fl oz) apple juice

About the Author

Kevin Finn graduated with a Bachelor of Science in Chemistry from Ohio University under the direction of Professor Mark McMills and received a Ph.D. in Organic Chemistry from Brock University in Ontario, Canada under the supervision of Professor Tomas Hudlicky. Following a Post-doctoral fellowship at Albert-Ludwigs Universität-Freiburg in Germany with Professor Dr. Reinhard Brückner, Finn returned to the US to pursue a career in pharmaceutical process development. He is currently employed in the Chicago area as a Project Manager and divides his spare time between studying martial arts and learning about- and promoting - juices for overall health. Kevin is indebted to his fiancée, Alexandra Dobrescu for the help, support and encouragement to see this work to completion. If you have questions or suggestions for new recipes, please post to https://canijuiceit.wordpress.com/ or write to kfinn.chemie@gmail.com

References

1 United States Department of Agriculture Scientific Report of the 2015
    Dietary Guidelines Advisory Committee: Advisory Report to the
    Secretary of Health and Human Services and the Secretary of
    Agriculture, February, 2015.
    http://www.health.gov/dietaryguidelines/2015-scientific-
    report/PDFs/Scientific-Report-of-the-2015-Dietary-Guidelines-
    Advisory-Committee.pdf

2 Merz, Beverly. "Micronutrients Have Major Impact on Health - Harvard
    Health." *Harvard Health Blog*, Harvard Health Publishing, Sept. 2016,
    www.health.harvard.edu/staying-healthy/micronutrients-have-
    major-impact-on-health.

3 USDA Agriculture Information Bulletin No. (AIB-792-2) November 2004,
Lin, B-H. ,Allshouse, J.E., Lucier, G. "U.S. Fruit and Vegetable
Consumption: Who, What, Where, and How Much"

4 United States Department of Agriculture, "Choose MyPlate." *Choose
    MyPlate*, www.choosemyplate.gov/.

5 USDA 2010 Report of the Dietary Guidelines Committee
http://www.cnpp.usda.gov/sites/default/files/dietary_guidelines_for_ameri
cans/2010DGACReport-camera-ready-Jan11-11.pdf, pages 1-453.

6 Reinagel, Monica. "Juicing: Healthy Habit or Blood Sugar Bomb?" *Quick
    and Dirty Tips*, 14 Aug. 2013, www.quickanddirtytips.com/health-
    fitness/healthy-eating/juicing-healthy-habit-or-blood-sugar-
    bomb?page=1.

7 Brandt, Michelle. "Little Evidence of Health Benefits from Organic Foods, Stanford Study Finds." *News Center*, 3 Sept. 2012, med.stanford.edu/news/all-news/2012/09/little-evidence-of-health-benefits-from-organic-foods-study-finds.html.

8 ; Bradman, A. et al. Effect of Organic Diet Intervention on Pesticide Exposures in Young Children Living in Low-Income Urban and Agricultural Communities *Children's Health*, **2015**, Vol. 123, 10.

9 Environmental Working Group. "Clean Fifteen™ Conventional Produce with the Least Pesticides." *EWG*, 2017, www.ewg.org/foodnews/clean-fifteen.php.

10 Environmental Working Group. "Dirty Dozen™ Fruits and Vegetables with the Most Pesticides." *EWG*, 2017, www.ewg.org/foodnews/dirty-dozen.php.

11 The Alpha-Tocopherol, Beta Carotene Cancer Prevention Study Group. The effects of vitamin E and beta carotene on the incidence of lung cancer and other cancers in male smokers. *N Engl J Med* **1994**; 330:1029-35

12 Jeukendrup, Asker. "Exercise Is the Best Antioxidant." *Jeukendrup - Trusted Sports Nutrition Advice & Exercise Science News*, Jeukendrup - Trusted Sports Nutrition Advice & Exercise Science News, 10 June 2018, www.mysportscience.com/single-post/2018/06/10/Exercise-is-the-best-antioxidant.

13 Calbom, C. *The Juice Lady's Remedies for Stress and Adrenal Failure*. Siloam, Charisma Media / Charisma House Book Group: Lake Mary, FL, 2014.

14 Kuzma, Cindy. "10 Perfect Post-Workout Smoothies." *Prevention*, Prevention, 25 May 2018, www.prevention.com/food-nutrition/recipes/g20452963/post-workout-smoothie-recipes/?slide=8.

15 Cross, J. *The Reboot with Joe juice diet: lose weight, get healthy and feel amazing*. Reboot Holdings, Pty Ltd. Austin TX, 2014.

16 Cross, Joe. "Joe Cross' 3-Day Weekend Juice Cleanse." *The Dr. Oz Show*, The Dr. Oz Show, 17 May 2018, www.doctoroz.com/article/joe-cross-3-day-weekend-juice-cleanse.

17 Varona, V. *Nature's Cancer Fighting Foods*, Page 53. Penguin Group (USA), LLC. New York, 2014.

18 Calbom, C. *The Juice Lady's Juicing for High-Level Wellness and Vibrant Good Looks*. Three Rivers Press, New York, 1999.

19 "Office of Dietary Supplements - Vitamin A." *NIH Office of Dietary Supplements*, U.S. Department of Health and Human Services, 2 Mar. 2018, ods.od.nih.gov/factsheets/VitaminA-HealthProfessional/.

20 Bonenberger, Marianne. "Chlorophyll." www.nature-education.org/chlorophyll.html.

21 Higdon, Jane, and Victoria Drake. "Chlorophyll and Chlorophyllin." *Linus Pauling Institute*, 1 Jan. 2018, lpi.oregonstate.edu/infocenter/phytochemicals/chlorophylls/.

22 "Chlorophyll." *Hippocrates Health Institute*, 1 June 2012,

hippocratesinst.org/well-being/chlorophyll.

23 Gomez Candela C, Bermejo Lopez LM, Loria Kohen V. Importance of a balanced omega 6/omega 3 ratio for the maintenance of health: nutritional recommendations. *Nutr. Hosp.* **2011** 26(2), 323–329 .

24 Adams P, Lawson S, Sanigorski A, Sinclair A. Arachidonic acid to eicosapentaenoic acid ratio in blood correlates positively with clinical symptoms of depression. *Lipids* **1996**, 31, S157–S161.

25 Hulett, V.L; Waybright, J.L. *Smoothies for Kidney Health: a Delicious Approach to the Prevention and Management of Kidney Problems & So Much More.* Kidney Steps, LLC, 2015.

26 "How to Add More Fiber to Your Diet." *Mayo Clinic,* Mayo Foundation for Medical Education and Research, 22 Sept. 2015, www.mayoclinic.org/healthy-lifestyle/nutrition-and-healthy-eating/in-depth/fiber/art-20043983.

27 Salamon, Maureen. "Are Fiber Supplements as Good as the Real Thing?" *LiveScience*, Purch, 29 July 2011, www.livescience.com/15302-high-fiber-diet-supplements.html.

28 Higdon, Jane, et al. "Magnesium." *Linus Pauling Institute*, 1 Jan. 2018, lpi.oregonstate.edu/mic/minerals/magnesium.

29 Kumar V, Sinha AK, Makkar HP, de Boeck G, Becker K. Dietary roles of non-starch polysaccharides in human nutrition: a review. *Crit Rev Food Sci Nutr.* **2012**; 52(10):899-935.

30 "E.hormone | Phytoestrogens." *E.hormone | Endocrine System : Types of*

Hormones, e.hormone.tulane.edu/learning/phytoestrogens.html.

31 Yildiz, F. *Phytoestrogens in Functional Foods*. Taylor & Francis Ltd. pp. 3–5, 210–211; 2005.

32 Tham DT, Gardner CD, Haskell, W.L.; Potential health benefits of dietary phytoestrogens: a review of the clinical, epidemiological, and mechanistic evidence. *J Clin Endocrinol Metab*. **1998**; 83(7):2223-2235.

33 Bloedon, Leanne T., Szapary, Philippe O. Flaxseed and Cardiovascular Risk. *Nutrition Reviews*, **2004**, 62(1): 18-27

34 Higdon, Jane, et al. "Vitamin C." *Linus Pauling Institute*, 8 July 2018, lpi.oregonstate.edu/infocenter/vitamins/vitaminC/.

35 Pawlowska, Edyta. "'Apple a Day' Advice Rooted in Science." *ScienceDaily*, ScienceDaily, 3 May 2011, www.sciencedaily.com/releases/2011/04/110412131923.htm.

36 Grotto, D. *101 Foods That Could Save Your Life!* Bantam Dell, A Division of Random House, Inc. New York, 2007.

37 Murray, M., Pizzorno, J., Pizzorno, L. *The Encyclopedia of Healing Foods*. Atria Books, New York, 2005.

38 Thomas , C. *50 Best Plants on the Planet*, Chronicle Books, Inc. San Francisco, 2013.

39 Reinhard, T. *Superfoods: the Healthiest Foods on the Planet*, Firefly Books (US), Inc. Buffalo, New York, 2010.

40 LD, Megan Ware RDN. "Cantaloupe: Health Benefits, Nutritional

Information." *Medical News Today,* MediLexicon International, 15 Aug. 2017, www.medicalnewstoday.com/articles/279176.php.

41 Wu K, Erdman JW Jr, Schwartz SJ, Platz EA, Leitzmann M, Clinton SK, DeGroff V, Willett WC, Giovannucci,E. Plasma and dietary carotenoids, and the risk of prostate cancer: a nested case-control study, *Cancer Epidemiol Biomarkers Prev,* **2004** Feb;13(2):260-9, Abstract, Accessed 13 December 2013.

42 Zhou, K., Raffoul, J.J. Potential Anticancer Properties of Grape Antioxidants; *J. Oncol.* **2012**, 8 pages.

43 University of Michigan Health System. "Benefit of grapes may be more than skin deep: Lower blood pressure, reduced heart damage." ScienceDaily. ScienceDaily, 23 April 2009.

44 Murray, M.T., *The Complete Book of Juicing,* Prima Publishing, Rocklin CA, 1997.

45 N. Kumar, A. Banik, P.K. Sharma. Use of Secondary Metabolite in Tuberculosis: A Review; *Der Pharma Chemica,* **2010**, 2 (6): 311-319.

46 Aviram M, Rosenblat M, Gaitini, D, et al. Pomegranate juice consumption for 3 years by patients with carotid artery stenosis reduces common carotid intima-media thickness, blood pressure and LDL oxidation. *Clin Nutr* **2004**;23 (3):423-33.

47 Biggs, M. *The Complete Book of Vegetables: the Ultimate Guide to Growing, Cooking and Eating Vegetables,* Firefly Books, 2010.

48 Castro-Torres, I.G., Naranjo-Rodríguez, E.B., Domínguez-Ortíz, M.A., Gallegos-Estudillo, J. and Saavedra-Vélez, M.V. Antilithiasic and Hypolipidaemic Effects of Raphanus sativus L. var. niger on Mice Fed with a Lithogenic Diet, *J. Biomed. Biotech.* **2012**, 2012, 161205.

49 "Benefits of Wheatgrass." *Hippocrates Health Institute*, hippocratesinst.org/wheatgrass/benefits-of-wheatgrass.

50 "Garlic." *Linus Pauling Institute*, 6 Jan. 2018, lpi.oregonstate.edu/infocenter/phytochemicals/garlic/.

51 Sharon, M., *The Complete Guide to Nutrients: An A-Z of Superfoods, Herbs, Vitamins, Minerals and Supplements*, 6th ed. Carlton Books, Ltd. London, 2014.

52 "Ginger." *National Center for Complementary and Integrative Health*, U.S. Department of Health and Human Services, 30 Nov. 2016, nccih.nih.gov/health/ginger.

53 Ellis, C. *Green Smoothie Joy, Recipes for Living Loving and Juicing Green,*. Skyhorse Publishing, New York, New York, 2013.

54 "Chimps, Humans 96 Percent the Same, Gene Study Finds." *National Geographic*, National Geographic Society, 15 Aug. 2018, news.nationalgeographic.com/news/2005/08/0831_050831_chimp_ge nes.html.

55 Mills, K. *The Green Smoothie Bible*, Ulysses Press. Berkley, CA, 2012.

56 Boutenko, V., Menzin, W.A., *Green for Life: The Updated Classic on Green Smoothie Nutrition*. Copyright North Atlantic Books, 2011.

57 Quillin, P., Quillin, N., *Beating Cancer with Nutrition*, Nutrition Times Press, Inc. Carlsbad, CA., 2005

58 Team, Wellness. "Recipe: Green Grape Smoothie." Health Essentials

from Cleveland Clinic, Health Essentials from Cleveland Clinic, 14 July 2015, health.clevelandclinic.org/2015/03/recipe-lucky-green-smoothie/.

59 https://minimalistbaker.com/coconut-clementine-green-smoothie/

60 https://minimalistbaker.com/

61 *"Dandelion Green Smoothie." Wholesomelicious, 27 Apr. 2018, www.wholesomelicious.com/dandelion-green-smoothie/.*

62 *"Crazy for Carrots." Simple Green Smoothies, 21 Feb. 2018, simplegreensmoothies.com/tips/carrots.*

63 Kennedy, T. *The Everything Giant Book of Juicing,* F+W Media, Avon MA, 2013.

64 *"Juicing Recipe: Creamsicle." Juice Recipes, juicerecipes.com/recipes/creamsicle-86.*

65 Calbom, C. *The Juice Lady's Guide to Juicing for Health,* M.S. Penguin Books, Ltd. New York, 2008,

66 Anderson, M. *Healing Cancer from the Inside Out.* www.RaveDiet.com, 2009.

67 "Homemade Baby Food Recipes - From First Foods to Full Meals." Homemade Baby Food Recipes To Help You Create A Healthy Menu For YOUR Baby, www.homemade-baby-food-recipes.com/.

68 "Smoothies for Babies & Toddlers." *Detoxinista,* 13 Nov. 2017,

detoxinista.com/smoothies-for-babies-toddlers/.

Made in the
USA
Monee, IL